Handbook of Obstetric Anaesthesia

A.S. Buchan and
G.H. Sharwood-Smith
Anaesthetic Department
Simpson Memorial Maternity Pavilion
Royal Infirmary of Edinburgh
Edinburgh, UK

W.B. Saunders
London   Philadelphia   Toronto   Sydney   Tokyo

W. B. Saunders   24–28 Oval Road
Baillière Tindall   London NW1 7DX

The Curtis Center
Independence Square West
Philadelphia, PA 19106–3399, USA

55 Horner Avenue
Toronto, Ontario M8Z 4X6
Canada

Harcourt Brace Jovanovich Group (Australia)
    Pty Ltd
30–52 Smidmore Street
Marrickville
NSW 2204, Australia

Harcourt Brace Jovanovich Japan Inc
Ichibancho Central Building
22–1 Ichibancho
Chiyoda-ku, Tokyo 102, Japan

©1991 W. B. Saunders Ltd

This book is printed on acid-free paper

Typset by Photographics, Honiton, Devon
Printed and bound in Great Britain

British Library Cataloguing in Publication Data is available

ISBN 0-7020-1540-7

Contents

Preface

An urgent summons to the labour ward may be viewed with apprehension by the anaesthetist. Prolapsed cord, massive maternal haemorrhage, eclampsia and the apnoeic baby are some of the emergencies which can be safely managed with a sound practical and theoretical knowledge of the basic procedures. This handbook, which is based on a manual produced for a large maternity hospital, is designed to meet this need.

The approach is of necessity didactic and we make no apology for this. The intention is to complement the excellent textbooks already available and we have selected a number of references which will enable the reader to develop an extended knowledge of current practice.

We hope that it will be a useful revision source for the practical element of postgraduate examinations and that more experienced anaesthetists will find it useful for the unexpected obstetric emergency.

Lack of communication between anaesthetist, obstetrician and midwife is regularly cited as a factor in maternal mortality and morbidity. Some of the areas covered, especially the resuscitation of mother and neonate, are common to the work of all three professional groups. It is therefore our hope that such a wider readership will find the handbook useful.

A.S. BUCHAN
G.H. SHARWOOD-SMITH

Acknowledgements

Several of our anaesthetic, obstetric and medical colleagues have given their valuable advice in the preparation of the book. We would particularly like to thank Dr A. Whitfield, Dr J.H. McClure, Professor A.A. Spence, Dr I.A. Greer, Dr I.A. Laing and Dr J.M. Steel for their assistance. We are especially grateful to Mrs Glynis Omond for typing the manuscript.

1 Physiological Changes in Pregnancy

CIRCULATORY CHANGES

Circulatory changes provide for the needs of the fetus and mother and also prepare the mother for blood loss at delivery.

Plasma volume increases by 45% while the red cell mass increases only by 20%. This results in the physiological anaemia of pregnancy (the haemoglobin falls from 15 g/dl to 12 g/dl at 34 weeks). The blood volume returns to normal 10–14 days postpartum (Fig. 1.1).

The systolic and diastolic blood pressures fall in mid-pregnancy then rise again to non-pregnant levels towards term, the diastolic showing a larger fall. In the last trimester changes in posture may have significant effects on the blood pressure. The central venous pressure shows no change during normal pregnancy. It should be noted that in labour the cardiac output will rise by 15% in the latent phase, 30% in the active phase and up to 45% in the expulsive phase.

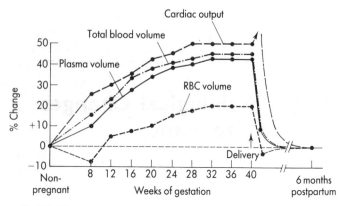

Fig. 1.1 Changes in cardiac output, plasma volume and red blood cell (RBC) volume during pregnancy and the puerperium (from Bonica, 1980).

Aortocaval occlusion

The gravid uterus, after 24 weeks, will compress the inferior vena cava (IVC) when supine causing a reduction in venous return and a fall in maternal cardiac output. Two compensatory mechanisms exist: first, there is an increase in sympathetic tone leading to vasoconstriction and an increase in heart rate; second, blood from the lower limbs may flow through the vertebral venous plexuses and via the azygos vein reach the right side of the heart. In 10% of mothers these mechanisms are inadequate to maintain a normal blood pressure when supine (supine hypotensive syndrome) and as the blood pressure falls consciousness may be lost. Turning the patient onto her side allows the blood pressure to return to normal as the inferior vena cava is decompressed. Falls in maternal blood pressure will lead to a reduced placental flow and the risk of fetal hypoxia.

Aortic occlusion frequently occurs simultaneously and leads to a decrease in blood flow to the kidneys, uterus, placenta and legs. This may again lead to inadequate placental perfusion and fetal hypoxia.

During labour these occlusive changes are exaggerated by the uterine contractions and most of the blood squeezed out of the uterus is forced into the extradural and azygos systems thus increasing extradural venous pressure.

Significance to the anaesthetist

Aortocaval occlusion. The induction of general anaesthesia or institution of an epidural or spinal are both procedures which will interfere with sympathetic tone and may therefore unmask aortocaval occlusion, leading to a fall in maternal blood pressure and placental perfusion. This must be anticipated and avoided by uterine displacement. During normal labour and delivery positioning of the patient is important to avoid aortocaval occlusion; this must not be forgotten at delivery, especially with forceps or ventouse.

Blood loss. At vaginal delivery this averages 300 ml and at Caesarean section 750 ml. This is well tolerated because of the increased blood volume.

Cardiac output. This increases immediately post-delivery due to auto-transfusion and improved venous return secondary to uterine emptying. Decompensation may occur in association with systemic or pulmonary hypertension, cardiac valvular disease and the use of vasopressors including ergometrine.

Epidural vein catheterisation. This is more common in the pregnant patient due to engorgement of epidural veins.

Utero-placental circulation

At term the uterine flow is 700 ml/min (10% of cardiac output) and some 80% of this will pass into the intervillous space via the maternal spiral arteries where exchange occurs between the villi containing the fetal capillaries and the maternal blood. Any reduction in the uterine blood flow will interfere with the transfer of nutrients across the placenta and must therefore be avoided if possible. Likely causes of reduced uterine blood flow are:

- *Hypotension*: IVC occlusion, blood loss, sympathetic block.
- *Hypertension*: essential or pregnancy-induced.
- *Uterine hypertonus*: excess oxytocin, placental abruption.
- *Vasoconstriction*: sympathetic overactivity due to fear/anxiety or sympathomimetic drugs (α-adrenergic) with the exception of ephedrine (mainly β-adrenergic).

RESPIRATORY CHANGES

The uterus displaces the diaphragm upwards. This is compensated for by an increase in both the anteroposterior and transverse diameters of the rib cage.

Alveolar ventilation increases by 70% in pregnancy, reaching its maximum at the second to third month of gestation. The changes in lung volumes and ventilation lead to a fall in P_aCO_2 to 32 mm Hg (4.3 kPa) and a rise of P_aO_2 to 105 mm Hg (14 kPa). There is no change in dead space, the oxygen consumption increases by 20% and the functional residual capacity (FRC) falls by 20%. In labour these values increase dramatically due to pain and anxiety (Table 1.1 and Fig. 1.2).

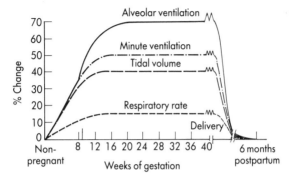

Fig. 1.2 Changes in ventilatory parameters during pregnancy (from Bonica, 1980).

Significance to the anaesthetist

An increase in capillary engorgement of the airway leads to swollen and easily traumatised mucosa. Airway obstruction occurs more readily with sedation and anaesthesia. The false cords swell and a smaller endotracheal tube may be required. These changes are exacerbated in severe pregnancy-induced hypertension. The changes in lung volumes and ventilation increase the efficiency of gas transfer to the benefit of the fetus but allow more rapid change to occur in maternal blood

Table 1.1 Changes in ventilatory parameters during labour may reach values of:

Respiratory rate	70/min
Tidal volume	2 litres
Minute ventilation	9–30 l/min
P_aCO_2	15–20 mm Hg (2–2.7 kPa)
P_aO_2	108 mm Hg (14.4 kPa)

gases than in the non-pregnant patient. This is seen especially with airway obstruction and on induction of general anaesthesia. Rapid falls in oxygen saturation occur due to:

(a) increased oxygen consumption at term;
(b) a fall in functional residual capacity;
(c) the fall in cardiac output in the supine position.

GASTROINTESTINAL CHANGES

Intra-abdominal pressure is increased and the axis of the stomach is altered, leading to delay in gastric emptying. There is an increase in fluid volume and a fall in gastric pH. The lower oesophageal sphincter pressure is considerably reduced—most pregnant women suffer from heartburn and some 30% have gastric reflux.

Significance to the anaesthetist

Obesity, multiple pregnancy, hydramnios and the lithotomy position will increase the likelihood of gastric reflux and possible pulmonary aspiration. Gastric acid with a pH of less than 2.5 is very irritant to the lungs and may lead to development of acute respiratory distress (Mendelson's syndrome). Narcotic analgesics given in labour significantly reduce gastric emptying and increase gastric volumes. Therefore, neutralisation of acid and a rapid sequence induction anaesthetic technique are mandatory.

RENAL CHANGES

Glomerular filtration rate and renal plasma flow increase rapidly in the first trimester and urine production increases. The clearances of urea, creatinine and urate are correspondingly increased and serum levels are below non-pregnant levels (Table 1.2).

There is increased aldosterone, progesterone and renin angiotensin activity. Consequently there is a rise in total body water and sodium. There is decreased reabsorptive capacity for glucose and lactose (glycosuria in 40% of pregnancies). Ureteric dilation is a progesterone effect, and associated urinary stasis may precipitate infection.

Significance to the anaesthetist

Renal problems encountered are usually in association with pregnancy-induced hypertension. Proteinuria occurs due to glomerular damage, oliguria may be a consequence of arteriolar damage and spasm which may lead to acute tubular necrosis.

HEPATIC CHANGES

Slight elevations in aspartate aminotransferase (AST), lactate dehydrogenase (LDH) and alkaline phosphatase are seen. Serum cholinesterase activity is reduced 25% at term and 33% three days postpartum. This is due to haemodilution and it is only in the postpartum period when the blood volume decreases that the duration of action of suxamethonium may be slightly increased by 2–3 min; this is not a clinical problem.

Table 1.2 Changes in renal function in pregnancy.

Investigation	Non-pregnant	Pregnant	Pathological in pregnancy
Plasma creatinine	73 μmol/l	50 μmol/l	>75 μmol/l
Plasma urea	4.3 mmol/l	2.3 mmol/l	>4.5 mmol/l
Plasma uric acid	0.2–0.35 mmol/l	0.15–0.2 mmol/l	>0.35 mmol/l
Plasma bicarbonate	22–26 mmol/l	18–22 mmol/l	
pH	7.40	7.44	

FURTHER READING

Bonica, J.J. (1980). Physiological changes in pregnancy. *In* "Obstetric Analgesia and Anesthesia", 2nd edn, pp. 1–24. Amsterdam: World Federation of Societies of Anesthesiologists.

2 Analgesia

PAIN PATHWAYS

Parturition pain

The pain of parturition is due to cervical and lower uterine segment dilatation, uterine contraction and distension of the structures surrounding the vagina and pelvic outlet. Initially the pain is felt in the lower abdomen but as labour progresses the distension of the birth canal by the descending part causes back, perineal and thigh pain.

Parturition pain pathways (Fig. 2.1)

Uterus and cervix. The afferent impulses are transmitted via the sympathetic nerves through hypogastric plexuses to enter the lumbar and lower thoracic parts of the sympathetic chain. Central connection to the spinal cord is by the white rami communicantes of T10 to L1. The pain of these contractions is therefore referred to the areas of skin supplied by these nerves in the lower abdomen, loins and lumbo-sacral region.

Vagina and pelvic outlet. The sensory nerve supply is

principally from the pudendal nerves (S2, 3, 4) with a minor contribution from the ilio-inguinal, genito-femoral and the perforating branch of the posterior cutaneous nerve of the thigh.

It is important to appreciate that pain-sensitive structures in the pelvis are also involved, i.e. the adnexi, the pelvic parietal peritoneum, bladder, urethra, rectum and the roots of the lumbar plexus. Therefore L2 to S5 must also be blocked. There is overlap and pain relief is not just a simple matter of blocking T10 to L1 for the first stage of labour and S2, 3, 4 for the second stage.

PSYCHOLOGICAL FACTORS

The threshold for requesting pain relief in labour is raised by antenatal preparation in the parentcraft classes. Education should be offered in the basic physiology of pregnancy and labour and there should be an emphasis on choice in analgesic methods. Relaxation and breathing exercises help the patient to control her perception of pain.

Anaesthetic interventions can be made easier and safer by reinforcing what has been taught in the parentcraft classes.

SYSTEMIC ANALGESIA

All analgesic drugs freely cross the placental barrier and narcotic drugs affect neurobehavioural responses in the neonate for up to 48 h. Pethidine is the most widely used systemic analgesic. The intramuscular dose is 50–150 mg and a single dose lasts for 2–3 h. Respiratory

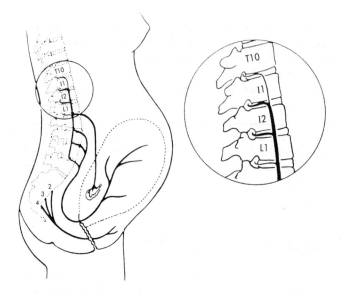

Fig. 2.1 Peripheral parturition pain pathways (from Bonica, J.J., 1980).

depression in the neonate is maximal when delivery occurs 3 h following administration. Unfortunately ineffective analgesia, nausea and dysphoria are frequent complaints. Morphine 5–10 mg and diamorphine 5–10 mg are more effective and longer acting. They have a greater potential for neonatal respiratory depression and are most useful in the primigravid patient when a longer labour is anticipated. The request for a second dose is an opportunity to consider the establishment of an epidural block. The problem of delayed gastric emptying is the most important maternal side effect with this group of drugs.

The agonist–antagonist group (pentazocine, butorphanol and nalbuphine) have the advantage of a ceiling effect for respiratory depression but ineffective analgesia and dysphoria are disadvantages. A further option is to use a patient controlled analgesia system (PCA). The anaesthetist can pre-set the incremental dose and minimum interdose interval.

Anxiety is best managed by the sympathetic support of partner or midwifery and medical staff. The use of benzodiazepine drugs should be a last resort because their use results in delayed fetal/neonatal metabolism leading to hypothermia and feeding difficulties. Nausea can be relieved by intramuscular cyclizine 50 mg or metoclopramide 10 mg.

TRANSCUTANEOUS ELECTRICAL NERVE STIMULATION

Transcutaneous electrical nerve stimulation (TENS) is an increasingly popular method of analgesia which is entirely patient controlled. Two lumbar and two sacral silicon rubber–carbon electrodes are applied by patient or partner and the amplitude and frequency are set to just above the sensory threshold. This may require some experimentation. At the onset of a contraction the patient can deliver a boost using a hand control. The method can be used as sole analgesia throughout labour and delivery. In general, however, it is more effective in the first stage than the second. It is important to emphasise to the patient that alternative methods of analgesia may be resorted to without any sense of failure.

By increasing large (A–β) fibre activity the hypothetical "gate" of Melzack and Wall is closed at a segmental level, thus reducing small fibre (A-δ and C) activity and therefore nociception. Full analgesia may not be achieved for 20 min or so. The range of controls used is typically:

current 0–50 mA, frequency 0–100 Hz and pulse width 0.1–0.5 ms.

INHALATION ANALGESIA

Entonox (50% nitrous oxide in oxygen) is self-adminis-tered from piped or cylinder supply by a facemask or mouthpiece and demand valve. It can either be used as a supplement to parenteral analgesia or alone from the onset of painful contractions in the first stage until the end of the second stage. Correct use is important and often neglected. The mask should be used with deep but slow respiration from the onset of a contraction before pain is experienced. Entonox is not inspired between contractions. Self-administration prevents excessive sedation. To avoid separation of the pre-mixed nitrous oxide and oxygen, cylinders should not be exposed to cold. If it is suspected that storage temperature has fallen to below −7°C the cylinder should be warmed to a safe temperature and inverted three times.

PARACERVICAL BLOCK (T10–L1)

To induce a paracervical block, 10 ml of 1% lignocaine or 0.25% bupivacaine are injected into each lateral fornix with a sheathed paracervical needle. This method of analgesia is associated with fetal bradycardia and acidosis and is rarely used nowadays. It may have a use for outpatient termination in early pregnancy, together with intravenous sedation.

PUDENDAL BLOCK (S1, 2, 3)

This is almost always done by the obstetrician. It is performed to relieve pain during the second stage of labour and provide anaesthesia for episiotomy and low forceps delivery. It is not adequate on its own for rotational forceps delivery but may be combined with inhalation anaesthetic agents, e.g. Entonox.

This may not give complete analgesia of the perineum because overlap may occur from the genital branch of the genito-femoral nerve and also the perforating branch of the posterior cutaneous nerve of thigh.

CAUDAL ANALGESIA IN OBSTETRICS

Indications

- Forceps delivery
- Pain relief in labour
- Suture of perineum

Caudals are rarely used now, but may be used in patients who have scoliosis or have had a spinal fusion. Veins in the caudal epidural space are engorged during pregnancy and the dose must be reduced correspondingly; for example, a volume of 30 ml will easily reach T9 in the pregnant patient.

Continuous caudals can be used but they suffer the disadvantage that large doses of drugs are needed to obtain pain relief in the first stage of labour and the catheter is in a potentially "dirty area". Caudals are not easy in the pregnant patient because the sacral hiatus is frequently obscured with a pad of fat. A useful method of ensuring that the needle is in the epidural space is to inject a small volume of air and listen with a stethoscope over the lumbar area. A crackling sound will be heard if the needle is in the correct position. In the second stage of labour a volume of 15–20 ml will give excellent pain relief.

The incidence of dural tap is much the same as with the lumbar approach. Intravascular injection may occur and penetration of the fetal head has been reported.

SPINAL ANALGESIA IN OBSTETRICS

Indications

- Cervical suture insertion
- Forceps delivery
- Caesarean section
- Manual removal of placenta, resuture of perineum, etc.

Advantages

- Quick onset of block
- Avoidance of general anaesthesia
- Excellent analgesia and muscle relaxation
- Minimum drug dosage
- Cheap

Disadvantages

- Hypotension with high blocks
- Headache (occurs in up to 10% of obstetric patients)
- A one-shot technique (consider a continuous technique with catheter)

Solutions available

Hyperbaric bupivacaine 0.5%. This is the best solution for use. A dose of 2 ml will give a good block to T10 and is therefore suitable for manual removal of placenta and rotational forceps delivery. The solution is hyperbaric, so leaving the patient in the sitting position will allow saddle anaesthesia to be established if this is required for perineal suture. For Caesarean section 2.5 ml will give a reliable block to T4 (see p. 29).

Hyperbaric lignocaine 5%. This is not readily available, but it can be useful as it has a rapid onset. However, it is rather unpredictable in spread. Dosage for Caesarean section is 1.5 ml in the lateral position. If the solution is injected when the patient is in the sitting position very low blocks will be obtained.

Isobaric bupivacaine 0.5%. This can be used but is less reliable than the heavy solution. The dose for Caesarean section is 3 ml in the lateral position; for forceps delivery 2–3 ml in the sitting position.

FURTHER READING

Harmer, M. T. Rosen, M. and Vickers, M.D. (1985). "Patient-controlled Analgesia". Oxford: Blackwell.

Morgan, B.M. (1987). Problems of analgesia in labour. *In* Morgan, B.M. (ed.), "Problems in Obstetric Anaesthesia", pp. 163–175. London: Wiley.

3 Epidural Analgesia in Labour

INDICATIONS
- Maternal request
- Prolonged and painful labour (often in primiparous patients)
- Malpresentation
- Anticipated or actual instrument delivery
- Trial of labour
- Pregnancy-induced hypertension
- Premature labour
- Diabetic labour
- Uncoordinated uterus/accelerated labour
- Multiple pregnancy
- Cardiac and respiratory disease

Administer with caution

Epidural analgesia should be administered with caution if any of the following apply:

Previous Caesarean section. Sudden analgesic failure may be due to uterine rupture. Extensive blockade must be avoided in order to demonstrate this important sign.

Central nervous system disorders. In multiple sclerosis there is no evidence that demyelination can be provoked by epidural analgesia. In cerebrovascular accident, porphyria and other rare conditions the pathophysiology should be discussed with a senior colleague and if necessary the relevant specialist before a decision is made.

Spinal deformity. Technical difficulty may increase the risk of dural puncture and careful assessment with spinal X-rays may be indicated.

CONTRAINDICATIONS
- Anticoagulant therapy
- Coagulopathy
- Hypovolaemic shock
- Local sepsis
- Objection by patient
- Raised intracranial pressure

SUGGESTED TECHNIQUE

A description of technique cannot replace practical experience with a senior colleague. A safe method should be selected and adhered to until confident and competent.

(1) Establish the indications for epidural anaesthesia and review the patient's relevant obstetric, medical and anaesthetic history.
(2) Explain procedure and obtain patient's informed verbal consent.
(3) Set up a reliable intravenous infusion of saline or Ringer Lactate with, at least, a 17 gauge intravenous catheter.

(4) Check that an ampoule of ephedrine 30 mg is immediately available.

(5) Record baseline blood pressure and pulse.

(6) Arrange patient either in the left lateral or sitting position according to preference.

(7) Scrub and gown-up.

(8) Site the epidural in the L2/3 or nearest convenient interspace using a saline or air loss of resistance technique.

(9) Measure the epidural space–skin distance.

(10) Insert the catheter 4–5 cm into the epidural space, withdraw the needle and withdraw the catheter to leave 2–3 cm in the space or until the meniscus in the catheter falls.

(11) Ensure that blood or cerebrospinal fluid (CSF) will not flow back either by capillary action or direct aspiration.

(12) Administer an epidural test dose 4 ml of 2% lignocaine. Inadvertent intravenous injection rapidly produces tinnitus and facial paraesthesia—enquire for this in a non-specific way to avoid suggestion.

(13) After 5 min record pulse and blood pressure and check for evidence of intrathecal placement (established sensory and motor blockade)—if in doubt wait and reassess after further 5 min.

(14) If test dose negative and blood pressure and fetal heart rate are stable administer bupivacaine 0.25% or 0.5% 5–8 ml.

(15) Progress over the next three contractions should indicate the efficacy of the block.

(16) Continue with top-ups or an epidural infusion according to preference.

PROBLEMS

Positive intravenous test dose.   Withdraw the catheter and resite in an adjacent interspace.

Failure to thread epidural catheter.   If associated with marked paraesthesia or failure of the following methods, resite in an adjacent interspace.

- Inject additional saline or lignocaine (3–6 ml) in an attempt to open up a plane.
- Carefully rotate the Tuohy needle through 180° (risk of dural tear). Do not withdraw the catheter through the needle (risk of dividing catheter).
- Ask the patient to extend her legs slowly.

Unilateral or patchy block

- Withdraw end-hole catheter to leave 1.5 cm in epidural space or 2 cm for side-hole.
- Use posture and the effect of gravity to help the spread of additional local anaesthetic.
- If these fail loculation due to epidural connective tissue is likely and the catheter should be resited.
- If a patchy block persists after resiting consider the addition of fentanyl 50 μg.

Patient is very obese

- Explain that the procedure may be difficult and use the sitting position.
- Identify the midline by palpating the upper thoracic spine.
- Palpate the iliac crest and draw a line bisecting the midline.
- Infiltrate subcutaneously for 5 cm above and below this point using 1% lignocaine.

- Use two or three 21 gauge needles to probe and mark this midline and a spine and interspace.
- If necessary use a long (15 cm) Tuohy needle.

Hypotension.   Initial symptoms are often due to the rate of fall rather than the absolute level of blood pressure. The complaint is of nausea, dizziness or sleepiness. Turn the patient onto her side (preferably left) to avoid aortocaval compression. Give 250 ml saline or Ringer Lactate rapidly and elevate the foot of the bed. In the absence of a rapid response ephedrine is administered intravenously in 5–10 mg increments until stability is restored.

Inadvertent dural puncture

- Resite the epidural in an adjacent space.
- Advise the obstetrician to consider a forceps delivery which will minimise CSF loss.
- Set up an epidural infusion of 1–1.5 litres Ringer Lactate over 24 h postpartum.
- Patient should remain in bed with one pillow for 12 h when she may sit up. If on completing the infusion the patient has no spinal headache she may slowly mobilise to normal activities; otherwise a dural blood patch should be recommended.
- Development of spinal headache is characterised by severe disabling fronto-occipital pain with radiation to neck and shoulders. There may be neck stiffness. The pain may be almost completely relieved by lying supine.

Management of spinal headache.   Discuss the nature of the problem and its management with the patient. If a blood patch is indicated it is commonly performed on the day following delivery. The procedure is as follows:

- A Tuohy needle is sited in the epidural space overlying the puncture site using a standard epidural technique.
- An assistant scrubs and gloves up to take 20 ml autologous blood under sterile conditions.
- 15–20 ml of the patient's own blood are injected slowly into the epidural space, stopping if it becomes uncomfortable.
- The patient lies flat for an hour and then slowly mobilises.

Conservative treatment of spinal headache is as follows:

- Encourage the patient to take oral fluids.
- Co-proxamol, dihydrocodeine or similar analgesia.
- Consider desmopressin (DDAVP) 4 μg intramuscularly twice daily for 3 days.
- Advise the patient that spontaneous resolution is likely within 3–5 days.

Subdural block

- Negative epidural test dose.
- After 5–15 min first main dose of local anaesthetic produces an extensive (to C7 or higher) sensory block with motor sparing (see p. 88).
- Distinguish from spinal block and if in doubt prepare to intubate and resuscitate patient.
- Manage hypotension in the standard way.
- If additional resuscitation is not required advise patient of likely rapid regression of block after one hour.
- If block regresses before delivery resite epidural (there is a risk of spinal penetration of the catheter and this may preclude the administration of a subdural top-up).
- Subdural catheter placement can be confirmed by

injection of radio-opaque dye in the postpartum period when the classic "tramline" appearance will appear on X-ray.

Total spinal block.   This is the subarachnoid injection of a large (epidural) dose of local anaesthetic. Equipment immediately required: resuscitation trolley with bag and mask; laryngoscope; endotracheal tubes; and suction pump.

- Position patient on left side.
- Administer oxygen with bag and mask.
- Call obstetric registrar and consultant anaesthetist as early as possible.
- Assistant performs cricoid pressure.
- Give 500 ml saline or Ringer Lactate rapidly intravenously.
- Give ephedrine 15 mg intravenously; repeat if necessary.
- Intubate patient if paralysis of respiratory muscles occurs.
- Use automated blood pressure and pulse oximeter monitors.
- Pass orogastric tube, empty stomach and instill 30 ml 0.3 molar sodium citrate.
- Maintain blood pressure with ephedrine and intravenous infusion until the block has regressed.
- Continually reassure patient.
- In the event of fetal distress delivery can take place when stable conditions are established.

EPIDURAL INFUSION

Following the establishment of an epidural block using the standard method described, a continuous infusion may be set up. There will be less risk of hypotensive episodes and an absent or infrequent need for top-ups. An 0.125% solution of bupivacaine run at 15 ml/h gives good analgesia. An 0.08% solution run at 20 ml/h will give a more extensive segmental spread with less motor block. Improved analgesia may be achieved by the addition of fentanyl to the infusion (see p. 101).

Recommended monitoring should include half-hourly blood pressure recordings, respiratory rate and upper sensory level testing. The infusion should be stopped and the anaesthetist informed if:

- Systolic blood pressure falls below 100 mm Hg.
- Skin numbness extends above the xiphisternum.
- Patient is unable to bend her knees or the weakness is getting worse.
- Infusion rate inaccurate.
- Respiratory rate falls below 9/min.

For methods of making up an infusion, see p. 100.

FURTHER READING

Covino, B.G. and Scott, D.B. (1985). "Handbook of Epidural Anaesthesia and Analgesia". Copenhagen: Schultz.

Gielen, M. (1989). Post dural puncture headache: a review. *Regional Anesthesia* **14**, 101–106.

Leading article (1987). Continuous extradural analgesia: catch-up or top-up. *Lancet* **ii**, 1300–1301.

Reynolds, F. (1989). Extradural opioids in labour (Leading article). *British Journal of Anaesthesia* **63**, 251–253.

4 Caesarean Section under Local Anaesthesia

EPIDURAL ANAESTHESIA FOR CAESAREAN SECTION

Prepare as for general anaesthesia.

Advantages

- The avoidance of the hazards of general anaesthesia (aspiration pneumonitis and failed intubation)
- Maternal and paternal participation in the birth
- Avoidance of drug-induced neonatal depression
- Good post-operative pain relief
- Improved bonding between mother and baby; early breast feeding

Disadvantages

- Maternal hypotension
- Length of time until onset of block
- Inadequate anaesthesia

Solutions available

The choice is between lignocaine 2% + 1:200 000 adrenaline and 0.5% bupivacaine with or without adrenaline.

The use of lignocaine on its own may lead to inadequate anaesthesia during the operation as the duration of action may only be of some 40 min. Lignocaine with adrenaline has a duration of action of the order of $1\frac{1}{2}$–2 h and is to be preferred.

Technique

One can either use an incremental technique or a single large volume injection. A single large volume technique does result in a better spread of local anaesthetic but there is the hazard of inadvertent intravenous injection, despite a negative test dose, which can result in convulsions and maternal death.

The incremental technique relies on the injection of small volumes of solution in increments, i.e. 5–7 ml. This can be varied with positioning of the patient from side to side or the injection may be made with the patient sitting and then with the patient lying down and moved from one side to the other.

These techniques all use injection through the catheter. There is another technique using injection directly through the needle which is claimed to avoid intravenous injection and the catheter is then passed after the main dose has been given.

The patients are given a fluid load of approximately one litre of Ringer Lactate. Colloids should be avoided because of the rare occurrence of anaphylactic reaction and consequent fetal hypoxia. An inflatable wedge is inserted under one of the patient's hips to ensure adequate tilting and avoidance of aortocaval compression.

During the onset of block hypotension is the main concern and the blood pressure must not be allowed to fall below 95–100 mm Hg systolic, otherwise inadequate placental flow may result in fetal hypoxia. Patients may complain of nausea or faintness and this should alert one to the possibility of hypotension. If this happens one must first ensure that the wedge is still properly in position. The patient can be tilted further onto her side, fluids should be infused and, if necessary, ephedrine should be injected, 7.5–10 mg intravenously. A block to T6 is required. To attain this height it may be necessary to give increments, alter the position of the patient, withdraw the catheter, etc. The level of skin analgesia must be tested, and if it is inadequate the patient should be offered the alternative of spinal or general anaesthesia for the operation.

A flow diagram for management of Caesarean section under epidural analgesia is shown in Fig. 4.1.

Management during the operation

The patient should be given a high flow of oxygen to breathe until the delivery of the infant. This ensures optimum fetal oxygenation in case there are problems extracting the child from the uterus. It is most important that a good rapport is established with the patient and maximum reassurance given. Once the operation has commenced it is usually only 5–10 min before the baby is delivered. After the baby is delivered the patient usually becomes far more relaxed, and previous complaints of discomfort may well disappear.

At the time of delivery oxytocin 5–10 units intravenously or 20 units into the infusion is given, the wedge is deflated and the oxygen may be discontinued.

Avoid the use of ergometrine as it usually results in nausea, vomiting and sometimes a considerable rise in blood pressure, which, in some patients, may precipitate left ventricular failure.

Management of inadequate block

(1) Plenty of reassurance.
(2) Nitrous oxide/oxygen (Entonox).
(3) Top-up the epidural.
(4) Intravenous opioid, e.g. fentanyl or diamorphine.
(5) 0.5–1% plain lignocaine may be injected or sprayed onto the peritoneum topically by the surgeon and this is often a valuable manoeuvre just prior to delivery.
(6) Induce general anaesthesia—this should not be delayed if the above measures are ineffective.

Post-operative analgesia

(1) Epidural opioids, e.g. 5 mg diamorphine with or without adrenaline in 10 ml of saline after delivery.
(2) Intramuscular opioids, e.g. 7.5–10 mg diamorphine intramuscularly 3–4 hourly.
(3) An epidural infusion of local anaesthetic, e.g. 0.125% bupivacaine. The efficacy of this can be improved with the addition of a small dose of opioid.

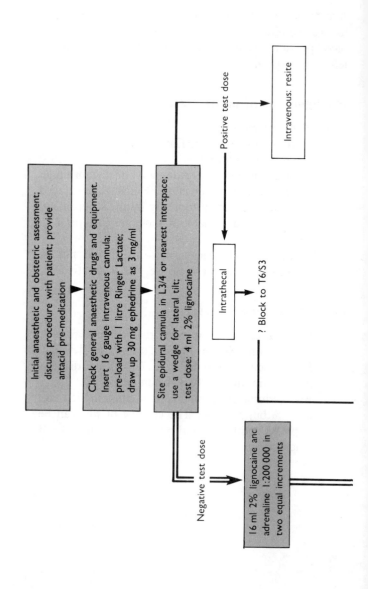

Initial anaesthetic and obstetric assessment; discuss procedure with patient; provide antacid pre-medication

Check general anaesthetic drugs and equipment. Insert 16 gauge intravenous cannula; pre-load with 1 litre Ringer Lactate; draw up 30 mg ephedrine as 3 mg/ml

Site epidural cannula in L3/4 or nearest interspace; use a wedge for lateral tilt; test dose: 4 ml 2% lignocaine

Positive test dose

Intravenous: resite

Intrathecal

? Block to T6/S3

Negative test dose

16 ml 2% lignocaine and adrenaline 1:200 000 in two equal increments

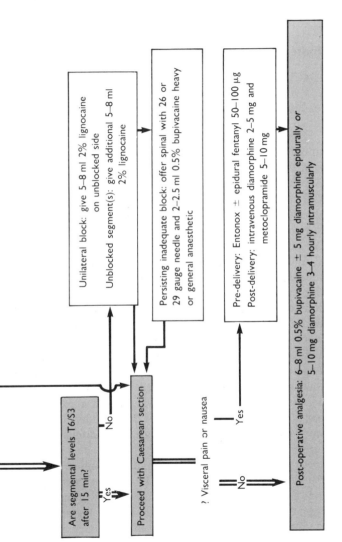

Are segmental levels T6/S3 after 15 min?

Yes → Proceed with Caesarean section

No →

Unilateral block: give 5–8 ml 2% lignocaine on unblocked side

Unblocked segment(s): give additional 5–8 ml 2% lignocaine

Persisting inadequate block: offer spinal with 26 or 29 gauge needle and 2–2.5 ml 0.5% bupivacaine heavy or general anaesthetic

? Visceral pain or nausea

Yes →

Pre-delivery: Entonox ± epidural fentanyl 50–100 µg

Post-delivery: intravenous diamorphine 2–5 mg and metoclopramide 5–10 mg

No →

Post-operative analgesia: 6–8 ml 0.5% bupivacaine ± 5 mg diamorphine epidurally or 5–10 mg diamorphine 3–4 hourly intramuscularly

Fig. 4.1 Management of Caesarian section under epidural anaesthesia.

SPINAL ANAESTHESIA FOR CAESAREAN SECTION

Indications

- Urgent delivery of infant
- Previous awake Caesarean section with inadequate analgesia

This should ideally be done with the 29 gauge needle to reduce the incidence of headache. This is most easily achieved with the patient in the sitting position. Aspiration with a clean 1 ml syringe will enable any CSF to be immediately identified. Injection is difficult through this needle and a good rigid introducer needle is essential to prevent hand tremor and displacement of the needle tip.

A dose of 2.5 ml of heavy bupivacaine will give a reliable block to T4. The onset of block with heavy bupivacaine 0.5% usually occurs within 5–10 min and consequently hypotension is likely. This is anticipated by infusing at least one litre of Ringer Lactate and it is worth considering the use of prophylactic ephedrine. Ephedrine should be drawn up ready for immediate use, or an ephedrine infusion may be preferred. It is essential that these patients are wedged properly to prevent aortocaval compression as this will, of course, exacerbate any hypotension. A pillow under the shoulders is helpful in preventing high spread. Oxygen is administered by face mask until delivery.

As spinal is a one-shot technique one must consider pain relief when it wears off. Intrathecal diamorphine 0.5–1 mg may be used and will give excellent analgesia. Monitoring respiratory rate for the first 12 h is advisable. If intramuscular opioids are used they must be given before the block wears off. Inadequate analgesia, hypotension, etc., must be treated as for epidural anaesthesia.

INFILTRATION ANAESTHESIA FOR CAESAREAN SECTION

It is important to know that Caesarean section can be done under local infiltration. This may be necessary if there are anaesthetic difficulties, no anaesthetist, or the poor medical condition of the patient may preclude anaesthesia. The visceral reflexes will not be abolished and complete pain relief is unlikely. Up to 100 ml of 0.5% prilocaine with adrenaline may be used (8 mg/kg maximum dose).

POST-CAESAREAN SECTION ANALGESIA WITH LOCAL ANAESTHETIC

Bilateral ilio-inguinal nerve block with bupivacaine

The ilio-inguinal and ilio-hypogastric nerves are blocked as they pass beneath the external oblique aponeurosis just medial to the anterior superior iliac spine. A dose of 10–15 ml of 0.25–0.5% bupivacaine is injected bilaterally. This will not give complete post-operative pain relief.

Local infiltration of the Caesarean section wound with bupivacaine

A total dose of 25 ml of 0.5% bupivacaine or 50 ml of 0.25% bupivacaine (2 mg/kg maximum dose) may be used. The muscle layer should be infiltrated after closure of the aponeurosis. Subcutaneous tissue should be infiltrated within $1-1\frac{1}{2}$ cm of the cut edge. Following infiltration there should be a degree of physical swelling of the subcutaneous tissue. If previous local anaesthetic has been given then this dose may need to be reduced.

EPIDURAL OPIOIDS IN OBSTETRICS

In the labouring woman epidural opioids do not completely remove the pains of labour. The addition of 50 µg of fentanyl to the initial bolus dose of bupivacaine will certainly increase its duration and efficacy.

There is a danger if one continues to use fentanyl throughout the first stage of labour that neonatal respiratory depression may occur.

Post-Caesarean section the use of opioids is of much more value in giving good pain relief. Diamorphine 5 mg in 10 ml of saline is the drug of choice. If it is combined with 1:200 000 adrenaline this will increase efficacy because less of the drug will be absorbed into the systemic circulation. It is wise to monitor the respiratory rate for up to 12 h after this injection although respiratory depression in young patients is extremely rare. Analgesia is normally good and will last for 8–12 h. The chief side effects are itching, nausea, vomiting and urinary retention. The itching and the urinary retention can be treated by giving intravenous naloxone. The advantages of epidural opioids post-operatively compared to bupivacaine are that one does not get motor block, nor does one have the problem of sympathetic block with subsequent hypotension. Intrathecally a dose of 0.5–1 mg of diamorphine is used. Side effects and indications are similar.

Policies vary but it is important to ensure that adequate parenteral analgesia is written up for these patients in case the expected long duration of the opioid does not occur. In the recovery period naloxone should always be at hand in case of respiratory depression. However, it is most unlikely that if patients are in pain they are really at risk of respiratory depression from subsequent opioid drugs.

Always use preservative-free solutions. There is no evidence of any nerve damage caused by intrathecal opioids.

FURTHER READING

Carrie, L.E.S. (1987). Regional techniques in obstetrics. *In* Wildsmith, J.A.W. and Armitage, E.N. (eds), "Principles and Practice of Regional Anaesthesia". pp. 112–126. Edinburgh: Churchill Livingstone.

Laishley, R.S. and Morgan, B.M. (1988). A single dose epidural technique for Caesarean section. *Anaesthesia* **43**, 100–103.

Moir, D.D. (1986). Local anaesthetic techniques in obstetrics. *British Journal of Anaesthesia* **58**, 747–759.

5 General Anaesthesia in Obstetrics

General anaesthesia is the third most common cause of maternal death in the United Kingdom. Mothers present particular difficulties because of:

- Presence of fetus and placenta
- Aortocaval compression
- Regurgitation and aspiration of gastric contents
- Intubation difficulties

PREPARATION FOR GENERAL ANAESTHESIA

A suggested antacid regime

Elective cases

- Ranitidine 150 mg orally at 22.00 h the night before
- Ranitidine 150 mg orally 2 h pre-op
- Local anaesthetic cream (EMLA) to intravenous site 2 h pre-op
- Sodium citrate 30 ml orally in the anaesthetic room

Emergency cases. Identify those at risk:

- Severe pre-eclampsia
- Abnormal presentation
- Multiple birth
- Antepartum haemorrhage
- Previous Caesarean section
- Trial of labour
- Fetal distress

A standing order will allow the midwife to administer ranitidine 50 mg intramuscularly to these patients.

Immediately the decision to operate is made, the following regime should be followed:

- Ranitidine 50 mg intravenously plus sodium citrate 30 ml orally
- Sodium citrate 30 ml orally is repeated in the anaesthetic room

Essential equipment

Suction machine, wedge, endotracheal tubes size 6 to 8 mm, an introducer (gum elastic bougie), two laryngoscopes (one with polio blade or short handle), oral and nasal airways, oesophageal gastric tube airway (EGTA), cricothyroidotomy set and laryngeal mask.

All these should be checked and laid out prior to induction of anaesthesia.

Monitoring equipment

Electrocardiogram (ECG), automatic blood pressure recorder, end tidal carbon dioxide monitor, pulse oximeter and peripheral nerve stimulator.

Drugs

Syringes of thiopentone 500 mg and suxamethonium 100 mg should be prepared daily, dated and stored in the fridge. An intravenous infusion should also be prepared daily and run through ready for immediate use. All drugs and intubation equipment must be renewed and checked by the anaesthetist who last used them in readiness for the next possible emergency.

Assistance

Two properly trained assistants should be present, one to perform cricoid pressure and the other to hand the anaesthetist the intubation equipment, etc.

INDUCTION OF GENERAL ANAESTHESIA

NEVER START WITHOUT ADEQUATE ASSIST-ANCE

- (a) Give sodium citrate 30 ml orally.
- (b) Wedge the patient to allow uterine displacement.
- (c) Switch on suction and place sucker under pillow.
- (d) Pre-oxygenate with 10 l/min for at least 3 min.
- (e) Administer thiopentone 250–350 mg (5 mg/kg) intravenously followed by suxamethonium 100 mg.
- (f) Cricoid pressure is applied as consciousness is lost and maintained until tracheal intubation and cuff inflation.

  CHECK POSITION OF ENDOTRACHEAL TUBE

- (g) Administer 50% nitrous oxide, 50% oxygen plus a volatile agent.

MAINTENANCE OF GENERAL ANAESTHESIA

(a) 50% nitrous oxide, 50% oxygen plus a volatile agent, either 0.5% halothane, 0.75% isoflurane or 1% enflurane.

(b) Administer a non-depolarising muscle relaxant, for example, atracurium 25–30 mg, once the suxamethonium wears off. If surgery is expected to be very rapid then one can use intermittent suxamethonium or a suxamethonium infusion after intravenous atropine. This is best monitored with a peripheral nerve stimulator. Avoid maternal hyperventilation; monitor end tidal CO_2.

(c) At delivery administer oxytocin 5–10 units intravenously as a bolus or add 10–20 units to the infusion, deepen anaesthesia with 5 mg diamorphine intravenously, reduce the inspired oxygen concentration to 33%, and deflate wedge. It is advisable to empty the stomach to reduce aspiration risk on awakening.

(d) Reverse any residual neuromuscular block at the end of anaesthesia, extubate the patient on her side with her awake after thorough suction of the pharynx.

(e) Move patient to recovery area.

FAILED INTUBATION DRILL

Every anaesthetist MUST have a drill to follow should intubation fail (see Fig. 5.1). Oxygenation is of prime importance—it is better to have a live patient with pulmonary aspiration than a patient dead from a hypoxic cardiac arrest.

(1) Decide urgency of delivery. Most cases can be

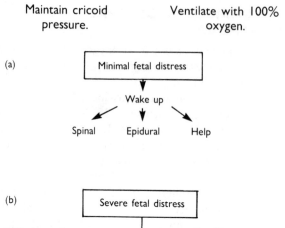

Maintain cricoid pressure.

Ventilate with 100% oxygen.

(a)

| Minimal fetal distress |

Wake up

Spinal   Epidural   Help

(b)

| Severe fetal distress |

Difficult ventilation

Easy Ventilation (maintain cricoid pressure)

Wake up

Cricothyroidotomy

Continue anaesthesia with a face or laryngeal mask

EGTA

Delivery

Spontaneous ventilation with N₂O/O₂ volatile agent

Spontaneous ventilation   IPPV

Empty stomach

Delivery   Delivery

Fig. 5.1 Failed intubation flow chart. It is essential to maintain cricoid pressure and ventilate with 100% oxygen.

allowed to wake up and either a spinal or epidural performed. Maintenance of cricoid pressure and ventilation with 100% oxygen are essential.

(2) Continue anaesthesia using a face mask with spontaneous ventilation N_2O/O_2/volatile agent. Maintain a clear airway with the help of oral and nasal airways and perhaps a laryngeal mask. This leaves the unresolved problem of a full stomach and continuous cricoid pressure may well make the airway difficult to keep unobstructed. Either a gastric tube can be passed, lifting off the face mask, or an oesophageal gastric tube airway (EGTA). This must be passed with the patient paralysed otherwise it will be difficult to insert and will result in vomiting. The stomach can then be emptied easily without interfering with the administration of the anaesthetic gases. A cuff inflated in the oesophagus will help prevent further regurgitation. If ventilation is easy then intermittent suxamethonium can be used.

(3) If ventilation with 100% oxygen is impossible a cricothyroidotomy using a cricothyroid puncture set or jet injection via a cannula will be necessary.

AVOIDANCE OF AWARENESS

Awareness, although rare in general anaesthesia, is more common in patients undergoing Caesarean section; this is because of the anxiety of the anaesthetist not to depress the baby. Awareness is to be avoided at all costs as almost all these women will suffer from severe postpartum depression. In addition awareness will lead to an overactive sympathetic system and an increase in catecholamine release, which may adversely affect placental flow.

Awareness may be avoided by:

(1) Using a large enough induction dose of thiopentone—4 mg/kg is certainly not adequate. Most cases of awareness are, in fact, vague memories of intubation.

(2) By the addition of sufficient volatile agents to 50% nitrous oxide/oxygen mixture. The recommended concentrations are up to 0.5% halothane, 1% enflurane and 0.75% isoflurane. Above these concentrations hypotension is more common and myometrial relaxation is more likely. If it is obvious that the mother is very lightly anaesthetised then one MUST INCREASE THE VOLATILE AGENT until one is sure that consciousness is lost. It is sometimes difficult to determine the depth of anaesthesia; most of the cases of awareness occur in patients having an elective Caesarean section who have had no previous opioids. The isolated forearm technique is a useful method of communicating with the patient during general anaesthesia for Caesarean section.

EMERGENCY CAESAREAN SECTION

The choice of general anaesthesia or local anaesthesia

All patients with fetal distress must be given 100% oxygen by face mask and transported to theatre in the lateral position to prevent further aortocaval occlusion and subsequent fetal hypoxia. Local anaesthesia will avoid many of the hazards of general anaesthesia, but remember it has its own hazards, especially hypotension, convulsions and apnoea. If an effective epidural is *in situ* then topping up to provide analgesia to T4 can be done with 2% lignocaine plus 1:200 000 adrenaline. This will act rapidly and the patient should be ready for Caesarean section within 5–10 min, depending on when the last top-up was given. If this has been more than 30–40 min ago then the dose really needs to be of the order 12–15 ml taking account of the analgesic level provided by the labour ward top-ups. Only very rarely should a patient with an adequate analgesic level be given a general anaesthetic for Caesarean section.

In dire emergencies a general anaesthetic may be necessary. Spinals are a very good way of avoiding the hazards associated with general anaesthesia if no epidural is *in situ* and delivery is relatively urgent.

ANAESTHESIA FOR MANUAL REMOVAL OF PLACENTA

Manual removal of the placenta can be done with general anaesthesia or local anaesthesia. If significant volume depletion has occurred due to blood loss or is expected during the procedure then local anaesthesia is contraindicated. If an effective epidural is *in situ* then a top-up to provide analgesia to T8/T9 is all that is required. A spinal is a good technique, but to avoid headaches a 29 gauge needle is preferred. General anaesthesia in all these patients should be with antacid cover, rapid sequence induction and intubation, avoiding excessive concentrations of volatile agents which may cause myometrial relaxation and further blood loss.

Occasionally it is necessary to give the patient 2–3%

halothane for uterine relaxation to allow the obstetrician access through the cervix to the placental bed.

ANAESTHESIA FOR *IN VITRO* FERTILISATION

In vitro fertilisation (IVF) involves laparoscopy for retrieval of ripened eggs and as it usually takes 30–40 min it is advisable to intubate and ventilate these patients. Because of the possible teratogenic effects of nitrous oxide a suggested technique is: thiopentone, atracurium, intubation, oxygen/enflurane/fentanyl with intermittent positive pressure ventilation (IPPV). The abdomen should be inflated with carbon dioxide rather than nitrous oxide.

ANAESTHESIA FOR CERVICAL SUTURE

Cervical suture procedure is usually done between 12 and 18 weeks gestation. Local anaesthesia such as spinal or epidural will reduce the number of drugs to which the developing fetus is exposed. General anaesthesia may be used quite safely with either a volatile agent or drugs such as fentanyl or alfentanil.

ANAESTHESIA FOR POSTPARTUM EVACUATION

Most patients with postpartum evacuation will present at least a week after date of delivery for evacuation of remaining uterine contents. It is probably safe enough to anaesthetise these patients with a mask, although again, consideration should be given to using both antacids and endotracheal intubation. The risks from regurgitation at this time are much less because the gravid uterus has been emptied, but nevertheless the physiological changes of pregnancy which have occurred at the lower oesophageal sphincter and in the gastric mucosa may not have returned to normal.

ANAESTHESIA IN THE PREGNANT PATIENT

Nitrous oxide has been shown to inhibit the activity of methionine synthetase, a vitamin B_{12} containing enzyme involved in DNA synthesis. There have, as yet, been no reports in humans of congenital anomalies associated with its use in the first trimester. Volatile anaesthetic agents in clinical dosage have not been shown to cause teratogenicity. It is the complications of anaesthesia, e.g. hypocarbia, hypercarbia and hypotension, etc., which are much more important factors as they will lead to reduced placental perfusion and fetal hypoxia.

Practical recommendations

(1) Only emergency surgery should be performed during pregnancy.
(2) Local anaesthesia should be considered.
(3) General anaesthesia in the first trimester—avoidance of nitrous oxide should be considered.
Second and third trimester—avoid aortocaval compression and remember to give antacids. Use a rapid sequence induction technique (see p. 38).
(4) Avoid hypotension, especially with epidurals and

spinals; ephedrine is the drug of choice; avoid hyperventilation; continuous monitoring of the fetal heart rate is recommended.

FURTHER READING

Fryer, J.M. (1987). Editorial. Anaesthesia for Caesarean section. *Hospital Update* **13**, 665–667.

Morgan, M. (1987). Anaesthetic contribution to maternal mortality. *British Journal of Anaesthesia* **59**, 842–855.

Thorburn, J. and Moir, D.D. (1987). Antacid therapy for emergency Caesarean section. *Anaesthesia* **42**, 352–355.

White, D.C. (1989). A review of nitrous oxide. *In* Atkinson, R.S. and Adams, A.P. (eds), "Recent Advances in Anaesthesia and Analgesia", vol. 16, pp. 19–42. Edinburgh: Churchill Livingstone.

Wilson, J. (1987). Problems of general anaesthesia in obstetrics. *In* Morgan, B. (ed.), "Problems in Obstetric Anaesthesia", pp. 1–9. London: John Wiley.

6 Complications of Pregnancy

PRE-TERM DELIVERY

Definition: Delivery prior to 37 weeks gestation.

Pre-term delivery, operative or by induction, may be indicated in intra-uterine growth retardation (IUGR), diabetes, pre-eclampsia or eclampsia. Pre-term labour may also be spontaneous.

Fetal immaturity, particularly of hepatic enzyme systems, means that conduction analgesia is preferable to opioids or general anaesthesia. An epidural established early in labour will facilitate a forceps delivery and can be maintained if necessary for a Caesarean section. The larger fluctuations in maternal blood pressure associated with the induction of spinal anaesthesia may prejudice placental intervillous flow and great care should be taken if this technique is chosen.

Tocolytic therapy

There are two pharmacological approaches to the management of pre-term labour. For longer term therapy a prostaglandin inhibitor may be indicated (e.g. indomethacin). In the acute situation a β-sympathomimetic agent is given. Ritodrine (predominantly a β-2 agonist) is frequently chosen and there are important cardiovascular and metabolic side effects with this group of drugs. These include maternal tachycardia, hypotension, fluid and sodium retention, hyperglycaemia, hypokalaemia and rarely pulmonary oedema.

Regional and general anaesthesia should if possible be avoided until maternal heart rate and blood pressure have been restored to close to baseline values. This normally occurs half an hour after halting the intravenous ritodrine.

HYPERTENSIVE DISORDERS

Pregnancy-induced hypertension (PIH)—pre-eclampsia/eclampsia

Definition: An increase in systolic pressure of more than 30 mm Hg and diastolic pressure of more than 20 mm Hg over the earliest pregnancy recording or an absolute reading of more than 140/90.

Generally the onset is after 20–24 weeks gestation and it should be distinguished from pre-existing hypertension on which pregnancy-induced hypertension may be superimposed. Serum urate is raised in proportion to the severity of the disorder.

Pre-eclampsia

- *Mild/moderate*: blood pressure over 140/90 mm Hg ± oedema.
- *Severe*: blood pressure over 140/90 mm Hg and significant proteinuria (> 0.3 g/24 h) or diastolic

blood pressure over 110 or cerebral disturbances, especially visual. The presentation may be pulmonary oedema.

Fulminating pre-eclampsia. Blood pressure is more than 180/120, there is usually oliguria and proteinuria, and there may be visual disturbance and headaches. This is a potentially life-threatening condition and cerebral haemorrhage, renal and hepatic failure and progression to eclampsia should be considered imminent.

Eclampsia. The prodromal signs in a patient with pre-eclampsia are severe headaches, epigastric pain, vomiting, visual disturbance and photophobia. Convulsions and coma can be expected to follow but can also occur without warning.

The multi-system nature of the disorder is such that some patients may present atypically with haemolysis, elevated liver enzymes and a low platelet count (HELLP syndrome). The rise in blood pressure may be unremarkable.

Oral anti-hypertensive drugs

These drugs are used to extend the gestation period as long as possible. This will allow fetal maturation by maintaining placental function and maternal organ perfusion.

- *Methyldopa*: in a dose of 1 g gradually rising to a maximum of 3 g daily in divided doses.
- *Labetalol*: in a dose of 100 mg rising to a maximum of 200 mg six-hourly.
- *Hydralazine*: in a dose of 25 mg rising to 75 mg six-hourly given alone or with methyldopa or labetalol.

- *Nifedipine*: initially in a dose of 10 mg three times a day.

Diuretics are generally not indicated since there is a reduced plasma volume.

In mild/moderate PIH a vaginal delivery is usually indicated. This is an indication for epidural analgesia which will help to control the blood pressure, increase placental perfusion, facilitate an instrumental delivery and avoid the exposure of a compromised fetus to opioids.

In severe PIH a coagulation screen should be obtained before siting the epidural. Do not site an epidural or spinal when there is a significantly abnormal screen and in particular a platelet count of less than 100×10^9/dl (avoid the use of adrenaline).

In fulminating pre-eclampsia the objectives are to control the hypertension, control or prevent convulsions, stabilise maternal haemodynamics and acid–base balance and deliver the infant as soon as possible.

There should be a controlled blood volume expansion using vasodilating drugs and intravenous fluids prior to general anaesthesia. Intensive monitoring of arterial and central venous pressure and urine output will avoid precipitating acute pulmonary oedema. Controlled oxygen should be administered and external stimuli such as noise and light should be minimised.

Obtain the following investigations: electrolytes, urea, creatinine, haemoglobin, liver function tests (LFTs), arterial blood gases, platelets and coagulation screen.

Convulsion management

Prevention

Chlormethiazole 0.8% infusion. This is run over

several minutes at 3 ml/min (60 drops/min standard giving set) until the patient is adequately sedated and then a maintenance infusion is given at about 1 ml/min (20 drops/min). However this may give rise to an excessive volume load, sedation and respiratory depression. Phenytoin is therefore preferred.

Phenytoin. The aim is to establish the therapeutic level of 10–15 μg/ml.

First dose	: Give 10 mg/kg in 100 ml normal saline at a rate of not more than 50 mg/min. Monitor respiration, pulse and blood pressure at 5-min intervals.
Second dose	: Give 5 mg/kg in the same way as the first dose 2 h later.
Maintenance dose	: 12 h following the second dose give 200 mg either orally or similarly to the regimes above intravenously.

The development of hypertension or arrhythmias such as heart block or sinus bradycardia is a possibility and it will be necessary to stop the infusion.

Treatment

Secure the airway and give oxygen. Diazepam 2.5–20 mg is given slowly intravenously. If this fails, thiopentone may be given in 25 mg increments intravenously only by an anaesthetist and intubation facilitated by suxamethonium may be required.

Blood pressure management

The objective is to control diastolic blood pressure at 100 mm Hg. In order to avoid cerebral ischaemia or placental hypoperfusion it is important not to exceed a fall of more than 25% of mean arterial pressure initially. Blood pressure and pulse should be monitored continuously.

Labetalol. 100 mg labetalol in 20 ml added to 80 ml normal saline (1 mg/ml). Start at a rate of 20 mg/h and double every 30 min to a maximum of 160 mg/h until the target blood pressure is achieved when the rate is kept constant. If bradycardia develops give atropine 0.6 mg and repeat as required. Asthma is a contraindication.

Hydralazine. Add 40 mg hydralazine to 500 ml normal saline (80 µg/ml). Start at 40 µg/min and double the rate every 30 min until the target blood pressure is attained. If severe maternal tachycardia develops use an alternative regime.

Rapid blood pressure reduction. Labetalol 50 mg intravenously over 2 min with 2-min recordings of blood pressure for 10 min reducing stepwise to half-hourly after one hour. This will take effect after 5 min and may last for up to 6 h. Alternatively, hydralazine 10 mg is given intravenously over 2 min with blood pressure monitoring as for labetalol.

General anaesthesia. All precautions and methods employed in standard obstetric anaesthesia are used (see p. 36). There is an added risk of difficult intubation due to laryngeal oedema. It may be beneficial to give 0.5 mg alfentanil or an increment of labetalol on induction to reduce the pressor response to intubation. For maintenance the vasodilating properties of isoflurane make it the preferred volatile agent with halothane as an alternative. Pass a nasogastric tube to empty the stomach before extubation since a prolonged period of deep sedation may be required post-operatively.

Post operative care. The patient should be transferred to the high dependency area. Anticonvulsant therapy should continue for 48 h or more and the hypotensive regime for as long as is necessary to maintain the target blood pressure. After 2 or 3 h a diuresis commonly occurs, but in the event of oliguria persisting intravenous frusemide may be required.

In the event of failure to stabilise the circulation and the development of pulmonary oedema or persistent oliguria it may be necessary to transfer the patient to the intensive care unit for the administration of trimetaphan/sodium nitroprusside (SNP) or dopamine. It is important to appreciate that pulmonary oedema develops as a result of left ventricular failure in the face of an excessive afterload imposed by systemic vasoconstriction. The pulmonary circulation is rarely affected as a primary event. Measurement of central venous pressure will give valuable information concerning the replacement of blood and fluids, but a realistic appraisal of left ventricular filling pressure will require the insertion of a pulmonary artery catheter.

MULTIPLE PREGNANCY

Twins

An effective epidural should be established early in labour. The anaesthetist should be in the labour ward during the second stage and the patient and equipment fully prepared for the administration of a general anaesthetic if required. Problems are most likely to occur with the delivery of the second twin and the aim should be for any instrumental or other obstetric manipulations or urgent Caesarean section to be conducted under an extension of the epidural block (see p. 42).

Triplets or quadruplets

There will be an increased risk of supine hypotension and regurgitation with aspiration due to the large uterus. Prematurity and pre-eclampsia are other hazards. Limitation of spinal flexion may lead to technical difficulties in siting a spinal or epidural; otherwise the management will be the same as for twins. Adequate equipment and staff will be required to resuscitate all the infants.

ANTEPARTUM HAEMORRHAGE

When there has been an antepartum haemorrhage (APH) the obstetrician may wish to do a vaginal examination to exclude placenta praevia. This must be performed in theatre where the patient and anaesthetist should be fully prepared for the immediate administration of a general anaesthetic in the event of a haemorrhage (see p. 61). Two units of cross-matched blood must be in the labour ward. When the placenta is not palpable the membranes are ruptured without anaesthesia and the patient is returned to the labour ward.

When there is a definite ultrasound diagnosis of placenta praevia an elective Caesarean section is performed at about 38 weeks gestation. The choice of regional or general anaesthesia will depend on the position of the placenta and the risk of haemorrhage at delivery.

PLACENTAL ABRUPTION

The management is determined by the clinical severity of the abruption. The condition may be complicated by a coagulopathy. The full extent of haemorrhage may not be revealed and if maternal hypovolaemic shock is apparent the procedure is as follows:

- A wide bore peripheral intravenous cannula should be sited in addition to a central venous line.
- A full coagulation screen is requested and repeated after a few hours if necessary.
- The procedure for management of major haemorrhage is followed (see p. 61).
- When haemodynamic stability has been established Caesarean section is performed under general anaesthesia.

DIABETES MELLITUS

The obstetric complications of diabetes mellitus include: polyhydramnios, macrosomia, pre-eclampsia and intra-uterine death. The neonate is at risk of hypoglycaemia. These problems have been reduced by "tight" antenatal control of maternal blood glucose levels. Antenatal monitoring of mother and fetus determine time and mode of delivery. An otherwise uncomplicated pregnancy will result in vaginal delivery at or near term. Oral hypoglycaemic drugs are not given in pregnancy.

The antenatal diabetic control is managed by the diabetic physician and obstetrician. However, in the event of a Caesarean section being indicated there must be close coordination with anaesthetic requirements. The anaesthetist must be able to take over diabetic management in the absence of a physician.

Caesarean section

Gestational diabetics not receiving insulin do not require any special management in labour. Insulin requirements are based on hourly blood glucose test strip estimations.

- An infusion of 500 ml of 5% glucose with 10 mmol potassium chloride is run at 125 ml/h and insulin is administered by a separate infusion pump typically at a rate of 0–3 units/h to maintain a blood glucose level at 4–9 mmol/l. Alternatively, the insulin can be added directly to the 5% glucose infusion.
- The patient should be encouraged to have epidural analgesia for either vaginal delivery or Caesarean section. This technique provides optimum conditions for the infant since opioids and other anaesthetic drugs will not be administered before delivery.
- An independent infusion should be sited for electrolytes, colloids or blood. Ringer Lactate should be avoided as it complicates the estimation of maternal carbohydrate load.
- Following placental delivery there is a rapid reduction in insulin requirement. The insulin infusion should be stopped and 5% glucose with 10 mmol potassium chloride continued at 125 ml/h until the blood glucose rises to 11 mmol/l. Insulin can then be restarted to maintain the desired blood glucose level, normally at 0–3 units/h.

Emergency

In this situation the management will depend on the current blood sugar level and the timing of the last insulin injection. If insulin has already been given and the patient is being starved 10% glucose is administered to give the equivalent in calories to the meal that is being omitted. If insulin is due then an infusion is set up as above.

Induced vaginal delivery

The following regime has proved satisfactory. The usual insulin is given the previous night and the usual breakfast is taken after only the short-acting insulin. A prostaglandin pessary is inserted in the morning and the situation reviewed at lunchtime. If labour is likely to become established lunch is omitted and an infusion of 5% glucose with 10 mmol potassium chloride is started and insulin is given according to the following sliding scale:

Blood glucose test strip: (mmol/l)

4 or less	no insulin
4–6	insulin at 1 unit/h
6–9	insulin at 1.5 units/h
9–11	insulin at 2 units/h
over 11	insulin at 3 units/h

A small number of patients may be insulin resistant, when up to 100 units/day may be required.

When labour is not likely to become established within the next 6 h lunch is taken and covered by short-acting insulin given subcutaneously.

Spontaneous vaginal delivery

As in the case of emergency Caesarean section the glucose and insulin requirements will be determined by the timing of the last meal and subcutaneous insulin administration.

RESPIRATORY DISORDERS

The normal maternal physiological changes (see p. 4) are required to maintain feto-maternal blood gases and hence fetal growth. The fetus is not often compromised by obstructive or restrictive disorders which will be severe if they have an adverse effect.

Sympathomimetic bronchodilators are given in the normal way as are inhaled steroids. Should systemic steroids be essential, additional cover will be required for both vaginal and operative delivery. In this case 100 mg hydrocortisone is given 6-hourly for 24 h followed by 100 mg 12-h for 48 h. Management will include antenatal respiratory function tests including blood gases when it is necessary to monitor progress closely.

Epidural analgesia is nearly always the technique of choice for obstructive or restrictive disorders. Severe scoliosis may present technical difficulties which should be anticipated and managed by adequate spinal X-rays. Optimum conditions may be provided by an elective forceps delivery.

CARDIAC DISORDERS

Cardiac disorders are managed on an individual basis by close liaison between anaesthetist, obstetrician and cardiologist. These problems are often complex and it is appropriate to give only general guidelines. Progress to term will be determined by the ability of maternal haemodynamics to adapt to the physiological requirements of pregnancy (see p. 1). The choice of anaesthetic technique demands a close study of the known effects of the method and drugs used on the cardiac disorder.

Normally the patient is not allowed to bear down for a vaginal delivery. In this case a cautiously administered selective epidural block will usually give the best conditions. Epidural anaesthesia will also help reduce preload after delivery when there is a sharp rise in cardiac output and an increased risk of pulmonary oedema. Pulmonary oedema at this time is treated with oxygen, intravenous opioids and frusemide.

Patients with cyanotic heart disease, such as Fallot's tetralogy or Eisenmenger's syndrome, are at risk of increased right-to-left shunt. This may be precipitated by the decreased systemic vascular resistance associated with an extended epidural block for Caesarean section. Regional analgesia may also be inappropriate when there has been a recent myocardial infarction. The fluctuating hypotension and arrhythmogenic potential of ephedrine are the precluding factors in this case. Elective Caesarean section in a well-sedated patient to whom a "cardiac" anaesthetic is given may provide optimum conditions.

Heparin therapy should be stopped before delivery and a coagulation screen should be normal before siting an epidural. Monitoring will be appropriate to the condition and may include pulmonary artery catheterisation and a radial artery line. In all cases it is essential that the patient is adequately oxygenated and is free from pain and anxiety.

FURTHER READING

Dailey, P.A. (1987). Anesthesia for preterm labour. *In* Shnider, S.M. and Levinson, G. (eds), "Anesthesia for Obstetrics", 2nd edn, pp. 243–262. Baltimore: Williams and Wilkins.

Greer, I.A. (1991). Hypertension. *In* Dunlop, W. and Calder, A.A. (eds), "High Risk Pregnancy". London: Butterworths.

Mangano, D.T. (1987). Anaesthesia for the pregnant cardiac

patient. *In* Shnider, S.M. and Levinson, G. (eds), "Anaesthesia for Obstetrics", 2nd edn, pp. 345–381. Baltimore: Williams and Wilkins.

Mudie, L.L. and Lewis, M. (1990). Pre-eclampsia its anaesthetic implications. *British Journal of Hospital Medicine* **431**, 297–300.

Ryan, G., Lange, I. R. and Naugler, M. A. (1989). Clinical experience with phenytoin prophylaxis in severe pre-eclampsia. *American Journal of Obstetrics and Gynecology* **161**, 1297–1304.

7 Major Obstetric Haemorrhage

Equipment must be available for measuring heart rate, ECG, central venous pressure (CVP) and intra-arterial blood pressure.

MANAGEMENT OF MAJOR OBSTETRIC HAEMORRHAGE

- Identify at risk patients.
- Summon senior help and extra staff.
- Alert haematology and blood transfusion staff.
- Anticipate coagulation problems.
- Stop source of haemorrhage.
- Insert two peripheral lines with large bore intravenous cannulae 14 g.
- Take 20 ml blood for cross-matching; order 10 units, preferably whole blood.
- Insert CVP line and display measurement.
- Infuse fluid rapidly with a pressure infusor and heating coil.

(a) Colloids until blood available (human albumin 4.5% is best) then gelatin solutions. Dextran 70—

only one litre should be given as it interferes with coagulation and cross-matching. Crystalloids are also necessary.

(b) Blood of the patient's own group is preferable. Group O Rh −ve in emergency uncross-matched patients except those who are known to have specific antibodies from the antenatal records. If more than 2 units of O Rh −ve blood have been given one must continue with O Rh −ve otherwise major intravascular haemolysis could occur due to increasing titres of transfused anti-A and anti-B antibodies.

(c) Do not give fresh frozen plasma (FFP), platelet concentrate or cryoprecipitate until major haemorrhage has ceased or until 6 units of stored blood have been given.

(d) Monitor pulse, BP, ECG, respiration, CVP, urine output and temperature. Check serially haemoglobin (Hb) or haematocrit.

(e) Consider drugs, e.g. calcium, bicarbonate, inotropes such as dopamine 2.5 µg/kg/min (see p. 100).

(f) Check blood gases and coagulation screen.

(g) Intensive care nursing.

(h) Prevent renal failure.

ANAESTHESIA IN CASES OF MAJOR OBSTETRIC HAEMORRHAGE

Frequently it is necessary to anaesthetise these patients in order to stop the source of blood loss. Obviously one must commence vigorous resuscitation before induction of anaesthesia but in many cases it is necessary to induce anaesthesia while resuscitation is in progress.

A rapid sequence of induction is used: pre-oxygenation, minimal doses of thiopentone, followed by suxamethonium and intubation together with cricoid pressure. Post-operatively these patients may require IPPV and if one has any doubts these patients should be transferred to the intensive care area.

ACUTE RENAL FAILURE

Diagnosis

Oliguria < 20 ml/h.

Pre-renal causes. Pre-renal causes of acute renal failure include hypotension and/or hypovalaemia, e.g. obstetric haemorrhage, hyperemesis, etc. The urine is:

(a) Concentrated, specific gravity > 1020; urine osmolality is high at > 700 mmol/kg.
(b) Low in sodium, the urine sodium concentration < 15 mmol/l.
(c) High in urea, the urinary urea concentration > 250 mmol/l.

The kidney is retaining maximum amounts of fluid and sodium.

Intrinsic renal causes. Acute renal failure may result from failure to correct pre-renal factors and/or exposure to nephrotoxins, e.g. bacteraemia, incompatible blood transfusion, disseminated intravascular coagulation (DIC), amniotic fluid embolus, cephalosporin and aminoglycoside antibiotics, non-steroidal anti-inflammatory drugs (NSAIDs) and hepatic failure. The urine is:

(a) Dilute, specific gravity < 1010; urine osmolality

is low at < 300 mmol/kg.
(b) High in sodium, the urine sodium concentration > 60 mmol/l.
(c) Low in urea, the urinary urea concentration < 160 mmol/l.

The kidney is not concentrating the urine effectively.

Management of oliguria

(a) Catheterise the bladder; measure hourly volumes; measure the urinary osmolality and sodium concentrations; obtain a specimen for culture and sensitivity.
(b) CVP monitoring.
(c) Correct hypovolaemia.
(d) Avoid nephrotoxins.
(e) Check electrolytes, full blood count and coagulation.
(f) If oliguria persists despite correcting pre-renal factors, then frusemide 40–80 mg intravenously is given and repeated as necessary. A low dose dopamine infusion may be indicated (2–5 µg/kg/min).

Management of renal failure

(a) Obtain advice/assistance from the renal unit at an early stage.
(b) Daily weight and fluid balance charts must be kept. Give 500 ml of 5% glucose plus the urine volume, blood loss and any naso-gastric aspiration.
(c) Monitor closely for hyperkalaemia. The urgent treatment of this is:

    (i)   10 ml of 10% calcium gluconate intra-venously.

    (ii)   500 ml of 5% glucose plus 10 units insulin intravenously.

    (iii) Sodium bicarbonate as necessary.

(d) The development of severe acidosis and hyperkalaemia are frequently an indication for dialysis.

COAGULATION PROBLEMS DURING PREGNANCY

The pregnant woman has a normal coagulation screen, the fibrinogen being at the upper limit of normal. Conditions predisposing to defective coagulation during pregnancy which require screening include:

- Shock from blood loss
- Severe placental abruption
- Amniotic fluid embolus
- Septic shock
- Severe pre-eclampsia or eclampsia
- Prolonged retention of dead fetus
- Incompatible blood transfusion
- Anticoagulant drugs, e.g. heparin.

Table 7.1 gives the normal range of values of coagulation parameters during pregnancy, and Fig. 7.1 illustrates the coagulation cascade.

USE OF ANTICOAGULANT THERAPY DURING PREGNANCY

Anticoagulant therapy is used during pregnancy to treat various conditions:

(a) Deep venous thrombosis (DVT) prophylaxis—heparin.

Table 7.1 Coagulation values.

Investigation	Normal pregnancy
Fibrinogen (g/l)	1.5–4.0
Platelets ($\times 10^9$/l)	150–400
Thrombin time (s)	15–20
Prothrombin time (s)	12–14
	therapeutic ratio: 2.0–4.0
Partial thromboplastin time (PTTK) (s)	35–40
	therapeutic ratio: control $\pm$ 6
Fibrin degradation products (FDP) (μg/l)	< 16
D-dimer (mg/l)	< 0.25

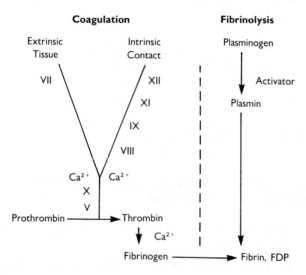

Fig. 7.1 Coagulation cascade.

(b) DVT treatment—warfarin.
(c) Prosthetic heart valve—warfarin.
(d) Antithrombin III deficiency—heparin.
(e) Pre-eclampsia—aspirin.

Oral anticoagulants

Vitamin K antagonists. Phenindione and warfarin. Warfarin has a low molecular weight, is lipid soluble, crosses the placenta and is teratogenic. It may cause prolonged bleeding, therefore change to heparin at 36 weeks. Laboratory monitoring is with the prothrombin time. Usually it is run at 2–3 times normal. Excess activity is treated with vitamin K.

Aspirin. Inhibits both vascular wall prostacyclin production (vasodilator, decreased platelet aggregation) as well as thromboxane A_2 production (vasoconstriction, increased platelet aggregation). It is thought that the thromboxane A_2 suppression is greater and of longer duration than that of prostacyclin suppression. So the net effect of aspirin leads to vasodilatation and decreased platelet aggregation.

Parenteral anticoagulants

Heparin. High molecular weight, does not cross placenta. Heparin inhibits a number of steps in the cascade which effect thrombin activity; it also influences platelet function. It is used widely in the later stages of pregnancy for DVT prophylaxis. Laboratory monitoring is with PTTK; usually it is 1.5–2.5 times the average control reading. Thrombin time can also be used but is much less sensitive.

Anticoagulants and epidurals

Heparin. Patients on heparin requesting epidurals should ideally have it stopped 12–24 h beforehand. The use of mini heparin is controversial. If the PTTK and platelets are normal, then it is probably safe to administer an epidural.

Aspirin. Chronic aspirin administration does affect platelet function but unless there is severe pre-eclampsia there seems little risk of haematoma formation if platelets are normal and bleeding time is less than 10.5 min. A coagulation screen should be obtained in moderate to severe pre-eclampsia in patients on aspirin therapy.

DISSEMINATED INTRAVASCULAR COAGULATION

Disseminated intravascular coagulation (DIC) is essentially a laboratory diagnosis with low levels of fibrinogen, factor V, factor VIII and platelets. There is evidence of enhanced fibrinolytic activity with high concentrations of fibrin degradation products (FDP). The FDP measure products from the fibrin monomer and fibrinogen. A new test, D-dimer, is specific for the breakdown products of the fibrin polymer, which is the basis of clot formation. Normally it is less than 0.25 mg/l. A high value would be in the range 8–32 mg/l. DIC coagulation values are given in Table 7.2.

DIC management

(1) Remove cause—shock, sepsis, hypoxia, empty uterus.
(2) Contact haematology department for advice.

(3) Repair haemostatic mechanism with FFP, cryoprecipitate, platelets. Heparin probably of little value; concentrates of antithrombin III may be useful.

Table 7.2 DIC coagulation values.

Investigation	DIC
Fibrinogen (g/l)	< 0.15
Platelets (× 10⁹/l)	< 50
Thrombin time (s)	> 100
Prothrombin time (s)	> 100
PTTK (s)	> 100
FDP (μg/l)	> 200
D-dimer (mg/l)	> 8

FURTHER READING

Guidelines for the Management of Massive Obstetric Haemorrhage (1989). Report on Confidential Enquiries into Maternal Deaths in England and Wales 1982–1984: pp. 29–30. London: HMSO.

Menon, D.K. (1989). Haemostasis in anaesthesia and intensive care (2). *In* Kaufman, L. (ed.), "Anaesthesia Review", vol. 6, pp. 105–116. Edinburgh: Churchill Livingstone.

8 Adult Resuscitation

CARDIOPULMONARY RESUSCITATION (CPR)

Basic CPR

*A*irway
*B*reathing
*C*irculation

After 26 weeks it is vital to avoid aortocaval obstruction by using a wedged board, otherwise external cardiac massage (ECM) will be ineffective as an empty heart is being compressed. If resuscitation is not successful after 2–3 min the baby must be delivered by immediate Caesarean section.

Advanced CPR

*D*rugs
*E*CG and defibrillation
*F*luids

Resuscitation drug dosages are given in Table 8.1 and Fig. 8.1 illustrates the procedures to follow to restore spontaneous circulation.

ANAPHYLACTIC SHOCK

Management

General resuscitative measures

- Airway
- Oxygen
- Intubation

Circulatory support with intravenous fluids and drugs.

Specific measures

Adrenaline	intramuscularly 0.5 ml 1:1000. intravenously 5 ml 1:10 000 slowly with ECG control.
Chlorpheniramine (Piriton)	10 mg intravenously (consider ranitidine 50 mg intravenously).
Hydrocortisone	100–200 mg intravenously.

If bronchospasm present:

Aminophylline	250–500 mg intravenously slowly.
Salbutamol	0.5 mg intramuscularly or 0.25 mg intravenously slowly. Nebulised, 2.5–5.0 mg in 3 ml saline.

Table 8.1 Resuscitation drug dosages.

Drugs (all doses based on a 70 kg woman)	Intravenous	Tracheal made up in a minimum volume of 10 ml NaCl	Comment
Adrenaline	1 ml 1:1000 (1 mg)	2 ml 1:1000 (2 mg)	Infusion 1 mg in 250 ml
Atropine	1 mg	2 mg	
Bretylium tosylate	500 mg	—	Slow injection, the agent of choice for bupivacaine induced cardiovascular dysfunction
Mexiletine	150 mg bolus	—	Infusion 1 gm in 500 ml

Calcium chloride	10 ml of 10%	—	Must not be injected with bicarbonate
Isoprenaline	100 μg	—	Infusion 2 mg in 500 ml
Lignocaine	100 mg	200 mg	Infusion 1.5 g in 500 ml (3 mg/ml)
Sodium bicarbonate	50 ml of 8.4%	—	Not as routine. Only refractory cases pH to be measured as soon as possible
Dexamethasone	10 mg	—	Follow with 4 mg intramuscularly 6 hourly
Dopamine hydrochloride	2.5 μg/kg/min	—	400 mg in 500 ml

Ventricular fibrillation (VF)

Monitor ECG

If flat trace check switches, connections and gain to ensure apparent asystole is not VF

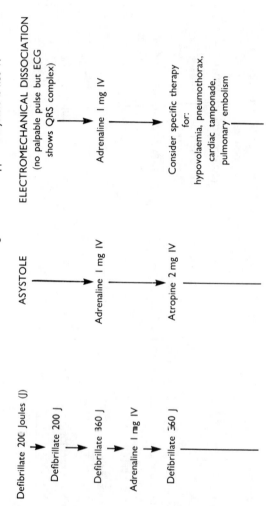

ASYSTOLE

ELECTROMECHANICAL DISSOCIATION
(no palpable pulse but ECG shows QRS complex)

Defibrillate 200 Joules (J)

↓

Defibrillate 200 J

↓

Defibrillate 360 J

↓

Adrenaline 1 mg IV

↓

Defibrillate 360 J

Adrenaline 1 mg IV

↓

Atropine 2 mg IV

Adrenaline 1 mg IV

↓

Consider specific therapy for:
hypovolaemia, pneumothorax, cardiac tamponade, pulmonary embolism

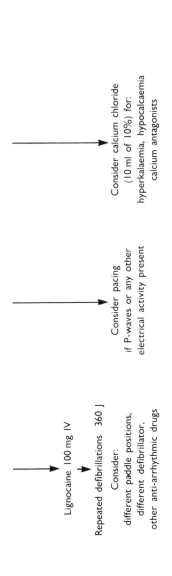

Lignocaine 100 mg IV

↓

Repeated defibrillations 360 J

Consider:
different paddle positions,
different defibrillator,
other anti-arrhythmic drugs

Consider pacing
if P-waves or any other
electrical activity present

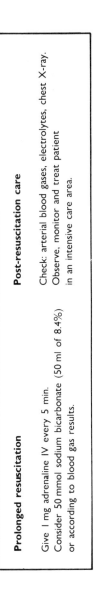

Consider calcium chloride
(10 ml of 10%) for:
hyperkalaemia, hypocalcaemia
calcium antagonists

Prolonged resuscitation

Give 1 mg adrenaline IV every 5 min.
Consider 50 mmol sodium bicarbonate (50 ml of 8.4%)
or according to blood gas results.

Post-resuscitation care

Check: arterial blood gases, electrolytes, chest X-ray.
Observe, monitor and treat patient
in an intensive care area.

Fig. 8.1. Restoration of spontaneous circulation (The Resuscitation Council UK, 1989).

AMNIOTIC FLUID EMBOLUS

Suspect in patients with sudden collapse or excess bleeding in labour or the immediate postpartum period. Predisposing factors include strong uterine contractions, uterine stimulants, uterine trauma, multiparity and premature placental separation.

Amniotic fluid embolus causes:

(a) Pulmonary vascular obstruction leading to a fall in left atrial pressure and cardiac output.
(b) Pulmonary hypertension leading to acute cor pulmonale.
(c) Gross ventilation perfusion inequality.

The four cardinal signs are:

- Respiratory distress
- Cyanosis
- Cardiovascular collapse
- Coma

They are frequently followed by disseminated intravascular coagulation (DIC).

Monitoring and treatment

(1) Intubate and ventilate with 100% oxygen consider positive end expiratory pressure (PEEP).

(2) If no pulse, then start external cardiac massage. AVOID AORTOCAVAL COMPRESSION.

(3) Insert two large peripheral cannulae, CVP line, urinary catheter, arterial line and if possible a pulmonary artery catheter.

(4) Aspirate blood from the right side of the heart for pathological examination (also check sputum).

(5) Monitor ECG, pulse, BP, CVP, pulmonary artery wedge pressure (PAWP).

(6) Draw blood for coagulation studies, cross-matching, arterial blood gases. Anticipate need for clotting factors.

(7) Deliver fetus and placenta as soon as possible.

(8) Drugs:

Isoprenaline	0.05–0.1 μg/kg/min (2 mg in 500 ml).
Dopamine	2–5 μg/kg/min (400 mg in 500 ml) (see p. 100)
Adrenaline	0.01 μg/kg/min (1 mg in 250 ml).

Calcium, sodium bicarbonate, frusemide, hydrocortisone, etc.

(9) Intensive care nursing.

(10) Treat DIC (see p. 68).

(11) Prevent renal failure (see p. 63).

CONVULSIONS

Main causes

Eclampsia, epilepsy and drug-induced. Consider all obstetric convulsions eclamptic in origin despite normal blood pressure until proved otherwise.

Premonitory signs

Eclampsia. May be NONE: severe headache (frontal) with visual disturbance; photophobia; nausea and vomiting and right upper quadrant pain.

Local anaesthesia. Subjectively: numbness of tongue and circumoral tissues; light-headedness; dizziness; difficulty focusing; tinnitus.

Objectively: slurred speech; shivering; muscle twitching.

Management

Turn patient on side to avoid caval compression. Maintain oxygenation and stop convulsions. Treat cause if applicable.

Diazepam	5–20 mg intravenously (more than 30 mg may cause neonatal hypotonia).
Phenytoin	10–15 mg/kg, slowly intravenously.
Chlormethiazole	0.8% solution, intravenous infusion.

Thiopentone, suxamethonium, intubation and IPPV.

MALIGNANT HYPERPYREXIA

Symptoms

(1) Tachycardia with or without ectopic beats.
(2) Tachypnoea.
(3) Raised temperature, rising by 2°C/h or more.
(4) An abnormal reaction to suxamethonium comprising rigidity.
(5) Rigidity developing later in the anaesthetic.
(6) Cyanosis.
(7) Increased oozing caused by development of DIC.

This diagnosis should be assumed if suspicions are aroused.

Signs

(1) Arterial desaturation ($Po_2 \downarrow$).
(2) Respiratory acidosis ($Pco_2 \uparrow$).
(3) Metabolic acidosis (pH $\downarrow$).

(4) Hyperkalaemia (K ↑).

Treatment

(1) Stop all anaesthetic agents immediately. CALL FOR HELP.
(2) Give 100% oxygen using IPPV with large minute volumes, i.e. 200 ml/kg.
(3) Stop surgery.
(4) Give dantrolene 1–3 mg/kg intravenously.
(5) Start active cooling with ice packs to major vessels and cold fluids intravenously.
(6) Correct metabolic acidosis with sodium bicarbonate 100 mmol.
(7) Monitor blood gases and pH.
(8) Monitor ECG, temperature, blood pressure, urine output.
(9) Take off blood for estimation of potassium level. Treat with dextrose and insulin if dangerously high.

FURTHER READING

Lee, M.D., Rodgers, B.D., White, L.M. *et al.* (1986). Cardiopulmonary resuscitation of pregnant women. *The American Journal of Medicine* **81**, 311–318.

Lessof, M.H. (1989). Anaphylaxis. *Prescribers Journal* **29**, 91–95.

Morgan, M. (1987). Amniotic fluid embolism. *In* Morgan, B. (ed.), "Problems in Obstetric Anaesthesia", pp. 121–138. London: John Wiley.

Rees, G.A.D. and Willis, B.A. (1988). Resuscitation in late pregnancy. *Anaesthesia* **43**, 347–349.

Safar, P. and Bircher, N. (1988). "Cardiopulmonary Cerebral Resuscitation", 3rd edn, London: W.B. Saunders.

9 Neonatal Resuscitation

PHYSIOLOGICAL CHANGES

At birth considerable changes occur to the neonate to allow adaptation to extrauterine life.

At birth the infant's first breath expands the lungs and reduces the pulmonary vascular resistance, thus allowing increased pulmonary blood flow. Clamping of the umbilical cord will cause an increase in systemic vascular resistance and these changes together with a rising arterial P_{O_2} result in closure of the foramen ovale and ductus arteriosus to establish a pulmonary and systemic circulation. The arterial P_{O_2} slowly increases and may take up to six weeks to reach adult values; this is due to increased intrapulmonary shunting which may be as high as 20% in the first few days of life. As the lungs expand more air accumulates, the surfactant function becomes well established and less negative pressure is required to allow air entry. Each subsequent breath therefore requires less effort.

Normally at birth blood from the umbilical artery has a pH of 7.25–7.22, a P_{CO_2} of 50 mm Hg (6.6 kPa), a P_{O_2} of 20 mm Hg (2.7 kPa) and a base excess of -5 to -8. Normal acid–base status is achieved after 1–2 h.

CHECKLIST PRIOR TO DELIVERY

(1) Switch on radiant warmer.
(2) Check oxygen supply and connections.
(3) Maximum pressure control blow-off is at 25 cm water.
(4) Suction apparatus functioning, oral mucus extractor and fine suction catheters, laryngoscopes, endotracheal tubes available.
(5) Dry and very warm towels available.
(6) Drugs ready: naloxone, adrenaline, dextrose and sodium bicarbonate.

NORMAL DELIVERY

Once nose and mouth are delivered suck out the mouth and oropharynx first and then the nose. This is because stimulation of the nose may cause the neonate to gasp and inhale the contents of the oropharynx. Be careful not to pass the sucker too far into the mouth as stimulation of the hypopharynx can cause laryngospasm and bradycardia.

As neonates have poor thermoregulation they should be dried and wrapped in warm towels. Most newborn babies do not need any resuscitation and after they have been dried they can be returned to their mothers.

ASSESSMENT OF THE NEONATE

Apgar score

The Apgar scoring system at 1 min and 5 min is in common use and gives information about the severity and prognosis of asphyxia.

Table 9.1 Apgar scoring system.

Clinical sign	Apgar score		
	0	1	2
A: Appearance (colour)	Blue, pale	Body pink, extremities blue	Completely pink
P: Pulse	Absent	Less than 100	More than 100
G: Grimace (reflex irritability)	No response	Grimaces	Cries
A: Activity (muscle tone)	Limp	Some flexion of extremities	Active, well flexed
R: Respiratory effort	Absent	Weak cry or shallow	Good strong cry

Score 10 = optimal condition.
Score 6 or less = depression; resuscitative measures required.

It has been suggested that an Apgar minus Colour Score (A − C) is better as colour does not correlate well with the acid/base state of the infant at birth.

The time taken from birth to the baby's first gasp and to the onset of regular respiration should be recorded.

ABNORMAL DELIVERY

Indications and management of the apnoeic baby (Fig. 9.1), meconium aspiration (Fig. 9.2) and acute blood loss (Fig. 9.3) are illustrated on the following pages [reproduced from "Resuscitation of the Newborn" (1988) Royal College of Obstetricians and Gynaecologists, with permission].

FURTHER READING

Resuscitation of the Newborn (1988). Working party of British Paediatric Association, Faculty of Anaesthetists Royal College of Surgeons England, Royal College of Midwives, Royal College of Obstetricians and Gynaecologists. Royal College of Obstetricians and Gynaecologists.

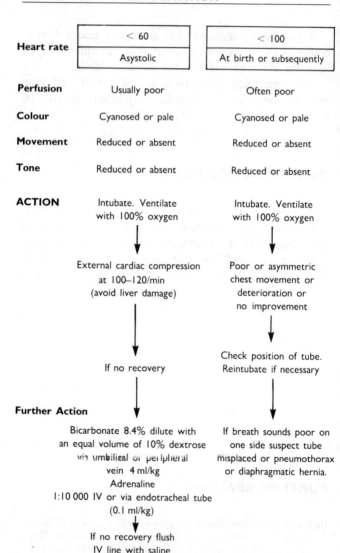

Heart rate	< 60	< 100
	Asystolic	At birth or subsequently
Perfusion	Usually poor	Often poor
Colour	Cyanosed or pale	Cyanosed or pale
Movement	Reduced or absent	Reduced or absent
Tone	Reduced or absent	Reduced or absent
ACTION	Intubate. Ventilate with 100% oxygen	Intubate. Ventilate with 100% oxygen

Intubate. Ventilate with 100% oxygen
↓
External cardiac compression at 100–120/min (avoid liver damage)
↓
If no recovery
↓

Intubate. Ventilate with 100% oxygen
↓
Poor or asymmetric chest movement or deterioration or no improvement
↓
Check position of tube. Reintubate if necessary
↓

Further Action

Bicarbonate 8.4% dilute with an equal volume of 10% dextrose via umbilical or peripheral vein 4 ml/kg
Adrenaline 1:10 000 IV or via endotracheal tube (0.1 ml/kg)
↓
If no recovery flush IV line with saline 0.9% and give 10% Ca gluconate 1–2 ml slowly.

If breath sounds poor on one side suspect tube misplaced or pneumothorax or diaphragmatic hernia.

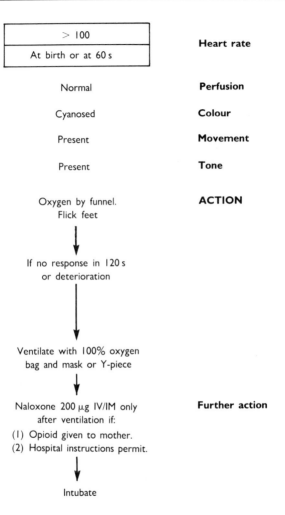

> 100
At birth or at 60 s

Heart rate

Normal   **Perfusion**

Cyanosed   **Colour**

Present   **Movement**

Present   **Tone**

Oxygen by funnel.   **ACTION**
Flick feet

↓

If no response in 120 s
or deterioration

↓

Ventilate with 100% oxygen
bag and mask or Y-piece

↓

Naloxone 200 μg IV/IM only   **Further action**
after ventilation if:
(1) Opioid given to mother.
(2) Hospital instructions permit.

↓

Intubate

Fig. 9.1 Indications and management of the apnoeic baby.

MECONIUM ASPIRATION

↓

Direct laryngoscopy

No meconium on or near larynx and baby well.

↓

Suction to oropharynx, posterior pharynx only.

Meconium distal to vocal cords.

↓

Intubate with largest tracheal tube possible (usually 3–3.5 mm).

↓

Aspirate meconium

With largest possible catheter   OR   Directly via the tube

If tube blocks

↓

Reintubate
Continue to aspirate until meconium is cleared.

↓

If condition deteriorates start IPPV using 100% O_2.

↓

Aspirate stomach with orogastric tube
before
transfer to Special Care Unit.

Fig. 9.2 Indications and management of meconium aspiration.

ACUTE BLOOD LOSS

Suspected prior to birth

e.g. ● Vasa Praevia
     ● Known fetomaternal
       bleeding

Unsuspected prior to birth

Signs including:

   ● Severe pallor
   ● Poor pulse volume
   ● Poor perfusion
   ● Tachycardia
   ● Inadequate ventilation

Immediate venous access
by umbilical catheter

Blood to laboratory for
haemoglobin, haematocrit
group, cross-match,
pH, and blood gases.

15 ml/kg of freshest
immediately available
Group 0 Rh −ve
blood. Give 5 ml/kg in
3 min followed by
remainder at a rate
dependent on speed of
improvement. Follow if
necessary with further
blood (use haemaccel
polyfusin, salt-free
albumin, or other volume
expander only if blood is
not available).

Fig. 9.3 Indications and management of acute blood loss.

Appendices

APPENDIX I:
ANATOMY OF THE SUBDURAL SPACE

Placement of an epidural catheter can occur in the subdural space between the dura and the arachnoid mater. This is a small potential space and a little drug goes a long way. Characteristically, injection of a small dose of local anaesthetic in this space results in delayed onset of a high sensory block usually not accompanied by motor block, nor by any significant hypotension. It is important that the differential diagnosis is made from subarachnoid injection by slow onset and usually lack of motor block. The anatomy of the coverings of the spinal cord help to explain the findings (see Fig. A.1).

On the dorsal nerve root there are separate attachments of the dura mater and the arachnoid, the arachnoid being fixed proximal to the ganglion and the dura distal. On the ventral root the dura and the arachnoid are attached together so that there is a potential space only over the dorsal root ganglion and pooling of local anaesthetic may occur at this point. If this is the case there is profound sensory loss with sparing of pre-ganglionic sympathetic fibres and the motor fibres carried in the ventral roots.

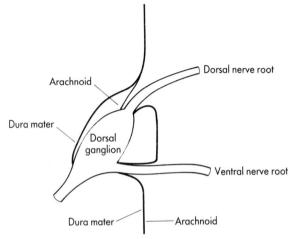

Fig. A.1 Dorsal nerve root ganglion with surrounding meninges. [Reproduced from Romanes, G.J. (ed) (1972) *Cunningham's Textbook of Anatomy*, 11th edition, Oxford University press, with permission].

The placement of a subdural catheter may, in fact, be responsible for the occasional case recorded of catheter migration, i.e. the catheter migrates through the arachnoid to the subarachnoid space and not through the much thicker dura mater.

APPENDIX 2:
USE OF ANTI-RH(D) IMMUNOGLOBULIN

Indications

(1) Rh(D) +ve infant born to Rh(D) −ve mother.
(2) If fetal cell count in maternal blood is raised (Kleihauer test).
(3) All Rh(D) −ve mothers for:
   • Termination of pregnancy

- Spontaneous abortion
- Threatened abortion
- Ectopic pregnancy
- Amniocentesis
- Antepartum haemorrhage
- Stillbirth
- External cephalic version for breech

Dose of anti-D

< 20 weeks—250 iu
> 20 weeks—500 iu

Supplies of anti-Rh(D) are dwindling as it is collected by plasmapheresis of sensitised women.

APPENDIX 3:
NORMAL CLINICAL CHEMISTRY VALUES

Investigation	Reference values
Acid/base measurements	
Hydrogen ion	36–44 nmol/l
P_{CO_2}	4.4–6.1 kPa
P_{O_2}	12–15 kPa
Plasma bicarbonate	21.0–27.5 mmol/l
Base excess	−4 – +4 mmol/l
Acid phosphatase	0.1–0.4 units/l
Alanine aminotransferase (ALT)	10–40 units/l
Albumin	36–47 g/l
Alkaline phosphatase	40–100 units/l
(Values in excess of 100 Units/l are often observed in childhood and adolescence and during pregnancy.)	
Amylase	50–300 units/l

cont'd

APPENDIX 3:
NORMAL CLINICAL CHEMISTRY VALUES (CONT'D)

Investigation	Reference values
Aspartate aminotransferase (AST)	10–35 units/l
Bilirubin (total)	2–17 μmol/l
Calcium	2.12–2.62 mmol/l
Chloride	95–107 mmol/l
Cholesterol (total)	3.6–6.7 mmol/l
Cholinesterase	0.6–1.4 units/l
	Dibucaine no. 77–83
	Fluoride no. 50–68
Creatinine kinase (CK)	30–200 units/l (M)
	30–150 units/l (F)
Creatinine	55–150 μmol/l
Electrolytes	
Potassium	3.3–4.7 mmol/l
Sodium	132–144 mmol/l
Total CO_2	24–30 mmol/l
Urea	2.5–6.6 mmol/l

Glucose	3.6–5.8 mmol/l
Liver function tests	
Alanine aminotransferase	10–40 units/l
Albumin	36–47 g/l
Alkaline phosphatase	40–100 units/l
Bilirubin	2–17 μmol/l
γ-Glutamyl transferase (GGT)	10–55 units/l (M)
	5–35 units/l (F)
Magnesium	0.75–1.0 mmol/l
Osmolality	280–290 mmol/kg
Oxygen saturation	Normally over 97%
Phosphate	0.8–1.4 mmol/l (fasting specimen)
Protein (total)	60–80 g/l
Urate	0.12–0.42 mmol/l (M)
	0.12–0.36 mmol/l (F)
Urea	2.5–6.6 mmol/l
Urea-stable lactate dehydrogenase (USLD)	100–300 units/l
Cerebrospinal fluid	
Glucose	2.5–4.0 mmol/l
Protein	100–400 mg/l

APPENDIX 4:
COMPOSITION OF BLOOD PRODUCTS AND COLLOID SOLUTIONS

Composition of blood products

Blood products	Vol/Pack	Contents	Remarks
Whole blood	450 ml + 63 ml CPD	Blood and plasma	Must be ABO + Rh(D) identical and cross-matched
Plasma reduced blood	300 ml	Concentrated red cells	Must be ABO + Rh(D) identical and cross-matched

Platelet concentrate	50 ml	Platelets	Must be ABO compatible
Fresh frozen plasma	180–200 ml	All clotting factors except platelets	Must be ABO compatible
Cryoprecipitate	20 ml	Factor VIIIc, fibrinogen, fibrinectin	ABO compatibility preferred
Plasma protein fraction (PPF)	400 ml	4.5% human albumin saline (no clotting factors)	Give to any blood group. Serious allergic reaction 1:30 000. Half-life is 16 days

APPENDIX 4:
COMPOSITION OF BLOOD PRODUCTS AND COLLOID SOLUTIONS (CONT'D)

Composition of colloid solutions

Colloid solutions	Contents	Plasma half-life	Serious allergic reaction	Remarks
Dextran 70	Glucose polymer	12 h	0.07%	Inhibits platelet aggregation and renders fibrin more susceptible to fibrinolytic enzymes. Take blood sample before use. Maximum volume 1–1.5 litres

Haemaccel	Polygeline (urea-linked)	5 h	0.14%	Contains 10 times more Ca and K than gelofusin. This may lead to clotting in heating coils when mixed with citrated blood or FFP
Gelofusin	Succinylated gelatine	4 h	0.06%	—
Hespan	Hetastarch	17 days	0.008%	Taken up by the reticuloendothelial system; final elimination from body very slow. Long-term effect of this is unknown

APPENDIX 5:
DERMATOME CHART AND SEGMENTAL NERVE SUPPLY TO THE PERINEUM

Dermatome chart

Skin area supplied by the dorsal nerve roots (Dermatomes) on the ventral surface of the body. Showing ophthalmic $\bar{V}1$, maxillary $\bar{V}2$ and mandibular $\bar{V}3$ divisions of the trigeminal nerve, the cervical, thoracic, lumbar and sacral nerves down to S3.

Segmented nerve supply to the perineum

Showing the skin area supplied by the sacral nerves 2–5 and the coccygeal nerve.

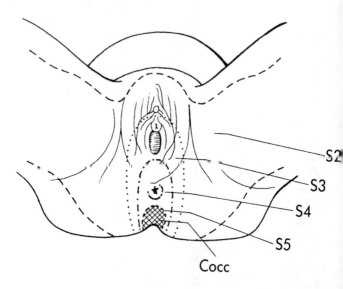

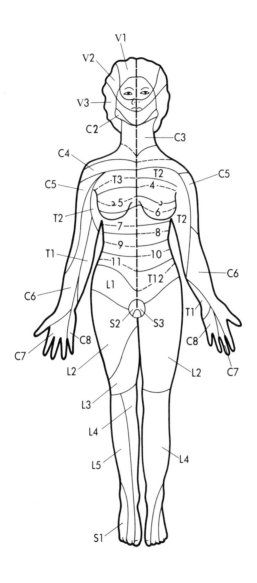

APPENDIX 6:
DOPAMINE

To make up a solution for a 66 kg woman

Take one ampoule of 200 mg dopamine and add it to 5% dextrose to make a total volume of 50 ml.

Run through an infusion pump, the setting of ml/h will equal dosage at rate of µg/kg/min.

Alternatively: Multiply the body weight in kg by 3 to obtain the dopamine dose, then add it to 5% dextrose to a total volume of 50 ml.

Run through an infusion pump, the setting of ml/hour will equal dosage at rate of µg/kg/min.

Different dosage regimes exert different effects:
2–5 µg/kg/min—predominantly renal effects.
5–10 µg/kg/min—predominantly β inotropic effects.
>10 µg/kg/min—predominantly α effects.

APPENDIX 7:
EPIDURAL INFUSION REGIMES FOR LABOUR

0.125% plain bupivacaine solution

(A) (1) Metriset with 120 ml "Buret".
    (2) 500 ml bag of 0.9% saline.
    (3) Place 30 ml of 0.5% plain bupivacaine in "Buret".
    (4) Add 90 ml of 0.9% saline to give 0.125% bupivacaine solution.

      (5) Establish epidural block, then administer solution at 15 ml/h.

(B) (1) 100 ml bag of 0.9% saline, remove 10 ml from it.

      (2) Add 30 ml of 0.5% plain bupivacaine.

      (3) Establish epidural block, then administer solution at 15 ml/h.

0.08% plain bupivacaine solution

(1) 250 ml bag of 0.9% saline, remove 40 ml from it.

(2) Add 40 ml of 0.5% plain bupivacaine to give 0.08% solution.

(3) Establish epidural block, then administer infusion at 20–25 ml/h.

Fentanyl may be added to the infusion to reduce the dose requirement for bupivacaine; at a rate of 15–30 μg/h. It is useful in enhancing perineal analgesia but pruritis may be a troublesome side effect.

Post-operative infusion regimes (volumetric pump)

0.125% plain bupivacaine solution: 500 ml bag of 0.9% saline; add 100 ml of 0.75% bupivacaine.

0.075% plain bupivacaine solution: 500 ml bag of 0.9% saline; remove 50 ml; add 50 ml of 0.75% bupivacaine. *Optional extra*: 20 30 mg diamorphine added to bag. *Infusion rate*: 8–15 ml/h, depending on height of block.

APPENDIX 8:
NORMAL HAEMATOLOGY VALUES

Investigation	Full-term infants	Adult female
White blood count ($\times 10^9$/l)	6.0–33.0	4.0–11.0
Red blood count ($\times 10^{12}$/l)	5.0–6.0	3.9–5.6
Haemoglobin (g/dl)	14.5–19.5	11.5–16.5
Haematocrit	0.44–0.64	0.35–0.47
Mean corpuscular volume (fl)	94–118	76–98
Mean corpuscular haemoglobin (pg)	32–40	27–32
Mean corpuscular haemoglobin concentration (g/dl)	34–36	30–35
Reticulolytes (%)	2.8–6.6	0–2.0
Platelets ($\times 10^9$/l)	100–400	150–400

APPENDIX 9:
REPORT ON CONFIDENTIAL ENQUIRIES INTO MATERNAL DEATHS IN ENGLAND AND WALES 1982–1984

Over the last 20 years the total number of maternal deaths from anaesthesia has decreased. However, the number of avoidable deaths has increased.

Maternal Anaesthetic Deaths

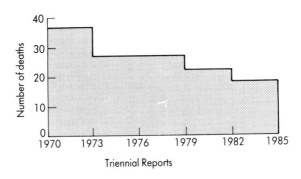

Fig. A.2 Maternal deaths from anaesthesia.

Causes of Direct Maternal Death

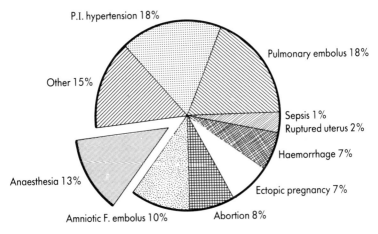

Fig. A.3 Causes of direct maternal death.

Table A.1 Contributing factors in maternal deaths 1982–1984.

Cause of death	Number	Contributing factors	
Endotracheal intubation problems	8	Oesophageal intubation	(4)
		Overinflated cuff	(1)
		Kinked tube	(1)
Inhalation of gastric contents	7	Substandard post-operative care	(3)
		Intubation difficulty	(2)
		Haemorrhage	(1)
Failure of adequate post-operative care	2	Inadequate neuromuscular reversal	
Apparatus misuse	1	Oxygen connection faulty	
Total spinal block	1	Epidural top-up by midwife, no anaesthetist in hospital	

The actual causes of death over the years have also changed and in this report anaesthesia was the third commonest cause of maternal death.

There were 19 deaths associated with anaesthesia in the 1982–1984 report, 18 directly and one in which anaesthesia made a contribution.

Conclusions

(1) Failure to intubate was cause of death in 10 patients.
(2) Checking position of endotracheal tube is essential.
(3) A failed intubation drill is essential.
(4) Inexperience of anaesthetists is invariably a factor.
(5) Better liaison between obstetric and anaesthetic staff prior to emergency surgery will reduce the incidence of problems.

APPENDIX 10:
NEUROLOGICAL DAMAGE FOLLOWING EPIDURAL/SPINAL BLOCKADE

Pathology	Cause	Onset	Clinical features	Outcome
Spinal nerve neuropathy	Trauma (needle, injection, catheter)	0–2 days	Pain during insertion, pain on injection, paraesthesia, pain and numbness over distribution of spinal nerve	Recovery 1–12 weeks
Anterior spinal artery syndrome	Hypotension Arteriosclerosis (use of adrenaline)	Immediate	Post-operative painless paraplegia. Posterior columns are preserved	Painless paraplegia

| Adhesive arachnoiditis | Irritant injectate | 0–7 days but may be much longer | May be pain on injection. A variable degree of neurological deficit often progressive with pain and paraplegia | Severe disability with pain and paralysis |
| Space occupying lesion (haematoma or abscess) | Coagulation defects bacteraemia | 0–2 days | Severe backache post-operatively with progressive paraplegia | Requires immediate surgery otherwise permanent paraplegia |

(From Covino, B.G. and Scott, D.B. (1985). "The Handbook of Epidural Anaesthesia and Analgesia". Copenhagen: Schultz.)

APPENDIX 11:
SIDE EFFECTS OF DRUGS ASSOCIATED WITH OBSTETRIC ANAESTHESIA

Drugs	Effect
Diuretics	
Ethacrynic acid	Neonatal deafness
Thiazides	Neonatal thrombocytopenia
β-Adrenoceptor blockers	Neonatal hypoglycaemia. Bradycardia and perhaps failure of the fetus to respond to hypoxia
β-Sympathomimetics	
Ritodrine (inhibits uterine activity in the short-term)	Maternal tachycardia, hyperglycaemia hypokalaemia, congestive cardiac failure and pulmonary oedema (especially with steroids)
Bronchodilators	
Terbutaline	
Salbutamol	May cause inhibition of labour with large doses

Antihypertensive drugs
Diazoxide
Nifedipine   May inhibit uterine activity
Verapamil
Sodium nitroprusside   Cyanide intoxication
Ganglion blockers
  Trimetaphan   Neonatal ileus
  Hexamethonium

Vasoconstrictors
Predominantly α-effects:
  Noradrenaline
  Metaraminol   May reduce placental perfusion
  Phenylephrine
  Methoxamine
Predominantly β-effects:
  Ephedrine   Will reverse hypotension due to sympathetic
  Mephenteramine   blockade without decreasing placental perfusion

cont'd

SIDE EFFECTS OF DRUGS ASSOCIATED WITH OBSTETRIC ANAESTHESIA (CONT'D)

Drugs	Effect
Anticoagulants	
Warfarin	Teratogenic, especially during first trimester. High incidence of haemorrhagic complications to mother and fetus. Do not use after 36 weeks
Heparin	Does not cross the placental barrier Safe
Barbiturates	
Thiopentone	Neonatal depression
Benzodiazepines	
Diazepam	Neonatal depression, hypotonia, hypothermia (bilirubin displacement from albumin by preservative sodium benzoate)

Narcotic analgesics	Intrauterine growth retardation with chronic abuse, intrauterine death with maternal withdrawal Neonatal depression Decrease in gastric emptying in labour
Non-steroidal anti-inflammatory drugs (NSAID) Indomethacin (prostaglandin inhibitor)	Inhibition of pre-term labour Premature ductus arteriosus closure
Aspirin	Prolongation of labour, increased incidence of haemorrhage in large doses
Anticonvulsants Phenytoin Carbamazepine Phenobarbitone	Congenital malformations. Enzyme induction leads to lowered vitamin K levels, neonatal bleeding tendency Vitamin K_I should be given to the mother at 36 weeks

cont'd

Drugs	Effect
Inhalation anaesthetics	
Halothane Enflurane Isoflurane Nitrous Oxide	Dose-related neonatal depression and myometrial relaxation, hypotension but no evidence of teratogenicity Interferes with DNA synthesis
[Operating Threatre Environment	Increase in spontaneous abortion and congenital abnormalities]
Local anaesthetics	
Prilocaine Lignocaine Bupivacaine	Methaemoglobinaemia > 600 mg (8 mg/kg) Large doses may cause maternal and neonatal depression especially after epidurals. Fetal bradycardia a feature after paracervical block Minimal neurobehavioural effects

Muscle relaxants

Quaternary ammonium compounds do not cross placental barrier in clinically significant amounts

Anticholinergics
Atropine

Fetal tachycardia and loss of beat to beat variation in large doses

Glycopyrrolate

Quaternary ammonium compound does not cross placental barrier

Oxytocic drugs
Oxytocin

Bolus dose can cause maternal hypotension due to vasodilatation

Excess may cause uterine hypertonia and fetal asphyxia

Ergometrine

Vasoconstriction occurs, hypertension

Pulmonary oedema

Corticosteroids

High doses cause maternal and neonatal adrenal suppression. Cover required during labour

APPENDIX 12:
WEIGHT CONVERSION CHART

Baby

Pounds (lb)	Kilogrammes (kg)
1	0.454
2	0.907
3	1.361
4	1.814
5	2.268
6	2.722
7	3.175
8	3.629
9	4.082
10	4.536
11	4.990
12	5.443

Adult

Stones	Kilogrammes (kg)
5	32
6	38
7	45
8	51
9	57
10	64
11	70
12	76
13	83
14	89
15	95
16	102
17	108
18	115
19	121
20	127

Index

Notes